ADVANCED DENTAL HISTOLOGY

A DENTAL PRACTITIONER HANDBOOK
SERIES EDITED BY DONALD D. DERRICK, D.D.S., L.D.S. R.C.S.

ADVANCED
DENTAL HISTOLOGY

W. A. GAUNT
M.SC. (Manch.), B.SC., PH.D. (Lond.)
Late Member of the External Scientific Staff,
Medical Research Council, London,
and Late Honorary Senior Lecturer in Special Anatomy,
Guy's Hospital Medical School, London

J. W. OSBORN
PH.D., B.D.S. (Lond.), F.D.S. R.C.S. (Eng.)
Reader in Anatomy in Relation to Dentistry,
Guy's Hospital Medical School, London

A. R. TEN CATE
B.SC., PH.D., B.D.S. (Lond.)
Professor and Chairman, Division of Biological Sciences,
Faculty of Dentistry, University of Toronto, Canada

SECOND EDITION REPRINT

BRISTOL: JOHN WRIGHT & SONS LTD.
1971

First Edition ('Advances in Dental Histology'), February, 1967
Second Edition ('Advanced Dental Histology'), June, 1971
Reprinted, August, 1972

ISBN 0 7236 0293 X

PRINTED IN GREAT BRITAIN BY
HENRY LING LTD., A SUBSIDIARY OF JOHN WRIGHT & SONS LTD.,
AT THE DORSET PRESS, DORCHESTER

PREFACE TO THE SECOND EDITION

As preparation of this second edition was about to begin, the sudden and untimely death of our colleague and friend Alwyn Gaunt occurred. We sincerely hope that his contribution has been revised for this edition as he would have wished. The rapid advances in the subject have necessitated complete revision and most of the chapters have been rewritten, the references expanded, and many of the diagrams are new or have been redrawn. Two new chapters have been added, one on collagen and the other on bone. In addition, a slight change has been made in the title of the book: *Advanced Dental Histology*, rather than *Advances in Dental Histology* is, we feel, a more accurate description of its contents, despite the fact that we do not intend to compete with specialized texts on single topics.

Finally one of us (A.R.T.C.) would like to acknowledge the help of Mrs. Karen Thiffault in the typing of part of the manuscript.

November, 1970
J.W.O.
A.R.T.C.

PREFACE TO THE FIRST EDITION

THIS book is not intended to be an orthodox textbook of dental histology but rather a supplement dealing with the latest, and often most controversial, aspects of the subject. Nor is it claimed that this book is fully comprehensive.

The rapid advances made in recent years in the field of dental histology involve the application of new disciplines, the results of which are to be found in an ever increasing range of scientific periodicals. In consequence, it has become increasingly difficult for students to find the time, and indeed the facilities, to collate this information from perusal of the original literature. Furthermore, the time lapse between completion of a manuscript and the appearance of a book is such as to preclude the incorporation of the latest information on any subject. It seemed to the authors, therefore, a worth-while service to review these latest advances, and to present them in a series of short essays in the least dogmatic manner. They are based upon the dental histology portion of the pre-clinical course given to students of dentistry at Guy's Hospital. Many of the ideas presented herein are still in the formative stage and may or may not come to fruition in the future. Nevertheless, they are included in the hope of providing a stimulus for further study and enquiry on the part of the reader.

If the rapid advances in this subject over the past few years continue in the future, it is anticipated that this book will require frequent revision if it is to be of continuing value. Realizing this, the book has been written so as to facilitate rapid revision by virtue of its simplified line diagrams and absence of photographic plates.

Every effort has been made to produce an authoritative book at low cost, consistent with the policy of constant revision. Rather than burden the reader with a long list of references to each chapter, only those which are readily available in most libraries are quoted, from which further specific references can be obtained.

February, 1967

W.A.G.

J.W.O.

A.R.T.C.

CONTENTS

ADVANCED DENTAL HISTOLOGY

CHAPTER I

THE INVESTIGATION OF TISSUES

THE aim of this chapter is to give an outline of the more important methods which are used to determine the structure and function of the dental tissues and to indicate a few of their limitations.

By far the most common tool used in the investigation of tissues is the light microscope, which in general requires the preparation of sections thin enough to transmit light. The preparation of thin sections of dental tissues necessitates either demineralization of hard tissues with the loss of the highly mineralized enamel or, if demineralization is to be avoided, the grinding of slices of dental tissue with the consequent loss of the soft tissue elements.

A wide variety of chemicals has been used to stain demineralized sections in order to make the thin, and therefore largely transparent, material visible under the light microscope. It is obvious that these stained sections appeared very different prior to being pickled (fixed), dehydrated, and wax-embedded, and yet most of our knowledge of the histological structure of the body, and much of our knowledge of how the body functions, has been learned by studying these stained remnants of the original tissue. The confidence with which interpretations are made is based on what is known as the 'reproducible artefact'.

It is of little value to mix together a number of chemicals and after staining a section with them to describe the appearance of the tissue in that one section. The proportions and concentrations of the materials and the time of staining must be carefully measured and controlled. The effect of using different proportions, concentrations, and staining times is studied and finally the combination which produces the best staining of tissue is selected. This type of experimenting is fundamental to light microscopy and many of the well-known staining procedures are named after the persons who originally formulated them (e.g., Mallory, van Gieson, Masson).

If a new tissue is to be studied, one or more of the well-known staining procedures is selected on the basis of the components of the tissues which are selectively stained by the method. The effects of the staining procedure are studied on a large number of sections until it is verified that the stain will always produce the same picture; in other words that the 'artefact is reproducible'.

Frequently we are interested in the overall appearance of a tissue rather than the minutiae of a single component contained within the tissue. One of the standard combinations of stains used for general histology is that of haematoxylin and eosin. Mature haematoxylin is a basic stain and there-fore attaches to acidic materials (e.g., the DNA and RNA of cells). Therefore nuclei are stained blue and cells rapidly synthesizing material (cells with a high proportion of RNA in the cytoplasm) will have a blueish cytoplasm. Eosin has an affinity for most materials and will stain all components red. It is therefore referred to as a 'counterstain'. Without this counterstain the material not stained by haematoxylin would be colourless and largely invisible.

For a more detailed study of some of the components of a tissue more selective staining procedures are required. Indeed, the value of a stain frequently depends on the specificity with which it will react with a com-ponent of a tissue. For example, certain silver solutions will precipitate on collagen, reticulin, and the axons of nerves. The brown and black artefacts produced by these precipitates may be reproducible but the value of sections stained in this way is often limited because of the difficulty in distinguishing which component of the tissue has been affected. Therefore, in the use of silver stains elaborate methods have been introduced in attempts to confine the precipitate to one specific component of the tissue.

Some of the most specific of staining techniques are those used in histochemistry. Histochemical techniques attempt to demonstrate microscopically the chemistry of cells and tissues. Such techniques usually depend on specific chemical reactions which form a coloured reaction product visible with the light microscope. An example illustrating the principles of histochemical practice is the simultaneous coupling azo-dye method for demonstrating the location of the enzyme acid phosphatase in tissue sections. The term 'acid phosphatase' is applied to the organic catalyst which, operating at an acid pH, splits phosphates from organic esters. Sections must be prepared without inactivating the enzyme or dislocating it from its intracellular position. In the case of the dental tissues this normally implies the cutting of unfixed, undemineralized frozen sections in order not to denature the enzyme. To such sections a solution is applied which is buffered at an acid pH (the working pH of the enzyme) and contains a substrate (sodium α-naphthyl phosphate) which the enzyme can split, together with a relatively colourless azo-dye. The enzyme splits the phosphate from the substrate exposing the naphthyl group which instantly combines with the azo-dye to produce a coloured reaction product at the site of the enzyme activity (*Fig.* 1). Using this method it is possible to demonstrate the activity of acid phosphatase in a wide variety of tissues.

It is sometimes helpful to view sections unstained. This is particularly true of the ground sections so commonly used in the study of dental tissues. In this case the picture seen under the microscope is produced due to differences between the light absorption, refractive indices, and optical interference of the component tissues. For instance, the dentinal tubules in a ground section are seen due to the difference of refractive index between the air contained in the tubule and that of the intertubular dentine. If the tubule becomes filled with calcified material, the tubule then has a similar refractive index to the intertubular material and the dentine becomes transparent. Probably the borders of enamel prisms are seen under the light microscope because of light reflection at the border separating adjacent prisms. The striae of Retzius appear brown by transmitted light because in the region of the striae blue light (shorter wavelength) is scattered away from the direction of viewing.

Frequently the optical heterogeneity of a specimen is difficult or impossible to see using the normal optical system of the light microscope.

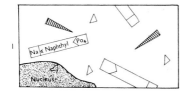

Diagrammatic appearance of section containing enzymes (cross-hatched) and nucleus (stippled). The section has been treated with sodium α naphthyl phosphate and azo-dye (triangle) in a buffered medium.

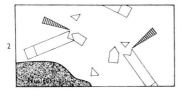

The enzyme splits off the PO_4- and the sodium α naphthyl component competes for the azo-dye.

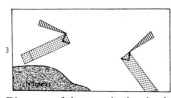

The PO_4- is replaced by the azo-dye to produce a coloured reaction product at the sites of enzyme activity.

Fig. 1.—Diagrams of the steps in the simultaneous coupling azo-dye method for demonstrating the location of the enzyme acid phosphatase in tissue section.

Phase contrast, interference, and polarization microscopy techniques use different optical systems to make these heterogeneities visible. For example, the phase contrast microscope will pick up very small, otherwise invisible, changes in refractive index.

Electron Microscopy.—The limit of resolution of the light microscope (the ability to distinguish two points as separate) is dependent upon the wavelength of light. Attempts have been made to improve resolution by utilizing radiations of shorter wavelength, such as X-rays, but the difficulty here is the inability to focus X-rays; hence at present X-ray microscopy is not a practical proposition. Far greater success has been achieved, however, by the use of electron beams which, although not part of the electro-magnetic spectrum, can be produced with a much shorter wavelength than light radiation. Also, as electrons are electrically charged, they can readily be focused by means of electro-magnets. The principles of electron microscopy are the same as for light microscopy (*Fig.* 2), except that electrons are used instead of light for illumination of the specimen and electro-magnets are substituted for the glass lenses of the light microscope. Because of the short wavelength, the resolving power of the electron microscope is over 100 times greater than that of the light microscope and true magnifications of up to × 1,000,000 are possible. The preparation of any tissues for electron microscopy is complicated by the fact that extremely thin sections are necessary as electrons have little penetrative power, and this raises additional technical problems so far as the dental hard tissues are concerned.

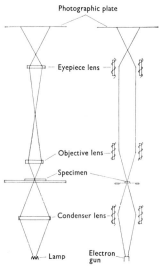

Fig. 2.—Diagram illustrating the similar principles
of light and electron microscopy.

Because the wavelengths of electron beams are outside the visible spectrum a black and white image of the tissue being examined is produced on a screen. Many cell organelles are bounded by lipids. These can be stained with the heavy metal in osmium tetroxide which absorbs electrons. On such electron micrographs the membranes will appear dark (they have absorbed electrons).

While the electron microscope has many advantages over the light microscope, the preparation and study of sections is very much more difficult. Therefore, whereas the cells studied by the light microscopist may be numbered in thousands, only a hundred may be studied by the electron microscopist. This poor sampling rate limits the value of electron microscopy. Furthermore, for many years much of electron microscopy was merely descriptive. For instance numerous types of vesicle have been described—coated vesicles, granular vesicles, dense vesicles, light vesicles, dark vesicles, and so on without much knowledge of the function of the vesicles described. It is only recently that sufficient knowledge of cell function has been acquired to enable functions to be allotted to many of the structures seen in electron micrographs of cells. Recently, histochemical and autoradiographic (*see below*) techniques have been used in electron microscopy. Such techniques have made it possible to interpret the function of some of the less obvious organelles seen by electron micro-scopists.

Both light and electron microscopes produce an image in two dimensions of what is substantially a two-dimensional slice of tissue. It is often difficult to visualize the appearance of the tissue in three dimensions.

In the scanning electron microscope a narrow beam of electrons is made to scan the surface of specially prepared tissues, rather like the spot on a television screen. The scanning beam is reflected from the surface of the tissue and ultimately on to a viewing screen. Because the beam obeys the normal laws of reflection an apparently three-dimensional image is produced of the surface scanned, based on the equivalent of light and shade. The image produced may be magnified up to 20,000 times. The scanning electron microscope has been used to investigate the precise shape of the mineralizing front in a wide variety of mammalian teeth.

Autoradiography is a more subtle form of identifying specific constituents in cells or tissues. In this instance, a substance used in normal metabolism (for instance calcium ions, an amino-acid, or a nucleic acid) is made

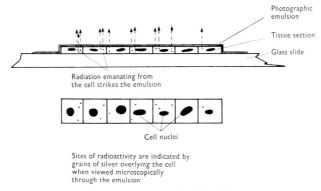

Fig. 3.—Diagram illustrating the principle of autoradiography.

radioactive and introduced into the living animal where it is utilized in an identical manner to its normal non-radioactive counterpart. Subsequently, this material can be traced in tissue sections due to its radioactivity. For instance, radioactive proline can be injected into a rat intraperitoneally. This proline circulates in the blood-stream and becomes utilized in the formation of collagen in the periodontal ligament. At a later date the animal is killed and sections of the periodontal ligament are prepared by normal histological methods. The sections are mounted on a slide and, in a dark room, are coated with a thin layer of photographic emulsion. After a few weeks in the dark room (the actual time depends on the half-life of the labelled atom) the emulsion is reduced over the spots where the radioactive proline is present. The emulsion is then developed photo-graphically and the section stained with haematoxylin and eosin. When the stained section is viewed through the now transparent emulsion, the silver grains indicate the exact spots where the radioactive proline has been incorporated (*Fig.* 3).

In one experiment the apices of continually growing rodent incisors were blocked with a filling material. Labelled calcium was now injected into the abdomens and a few weeks later the animals were killed. Ground sections of the incisors were cut and covered with photographic emulsion in a dark room. Subsequently it was observed that radioactive calcium had been incorporated in the newly formed enamel. Because the pulp cavity had previously been blocked, it is evident that the calcium must have come from the ameloblasts via the blood-stream proving that the enamel organ and not the pulp provided the mineral for enamel.

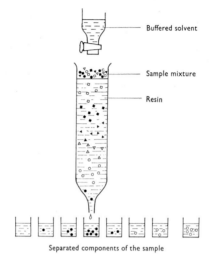

Buffered solvent

Sample mixture

Resin

Separated components of the sample

Fig. 4.—The principle of column chromatography.

The above methods can all give information on structure, and the newest electron microscopes may be able to resolve atoms. But the identification of composition at the level of atoms and molecules can only be undertaken by chemical techniques.

Every protein has three levels of structure which can be analysed: the proportion of the amino-acids it contains, the order of these amino-acids in the protein chain, and lastly the three-dimensional arrangement of the resulting chain or chains. Of these levels of structure the first (the proportion of the amino-acids) is the most easy to study while the second and third are extremely difficult and not often attempted.

It is not difficult to break the peptide bonds in a protein chain, thereby reducing the protein to its constituent amino-acids. In order to analyse the proportion of these amino-acids chromatographic techniques are used. Several methods exist but the principle involved is the same. A mixture of substances is made to move through a network or filter which differentially retards those substances that have, for example, a higher molecular weight or a positive charge. For instance, in column chromatography the sample to be analysed is washed through a long column of resinous material. The resinous material may be chosen preferentially to retard positively charged amino-acids and also have a pore size which will slow down the rate of movement of all the larger amino-acids. The amino-acids pass through the column at different rates (according to their size and charge) and can be collected separately at the bottom of the column (*Fig.* 4). Subsequently the proportions of each amino-acid can be determined. The data is usually given as numbers of amino-acids per 1000 residues. For instance, collagen in human dentine has 319 glycine molecules in every 1000 amino-acids, i.e., the collagen contains about one-third glycine.

Microradiographic Methods.—X-rays have a common application in the study of dental tissues. Most readers will be familiar with the conventional radiographs used in diagnostic medicine. Such radiographs rely on the use of X-rays generated at high voltage and of short wavelength, the so-called 'hard' X-rays. The same principle is involved with contact microradiography. The specimen is placed in contact with a recording photographic emulsion and exposed to 'soft' X-rays, generated at low voltages and of longer wavelengths. The X-rays are differentially absorbed by the specimen, depending on the number, the kind of atoms, and their capacity to absorb X-rays. From the resulting photographic record information can be gained about the overall pattern, degree, and detail of mineralization. For instance, peritubular dentine can easily be recognized using microradiography.

Experimental Methods.—Such methods usually depend upon altering the environment of the living tissue being studied in a specific way and observing any response with many of the techniques already described. Included in this category are experimental methods such as those designed to reveal the effect of specific dietary deficiencies and additions, ablation studies, and tissue culture studies. There are many other techniques in this category which have been used to investigate the dental tissues. Examples will be referred to in later chapters.

CHAPTER II

THE CELL

THE cell is the structural and functional unit of the living organism. Unicellular organisms have existed from the time of first life on earth and have colonized all known ecological niches. They must therefore be regarded as being highly 'successful'. However, it is the multicellular organisms that have provided the 'plastic' substrate upon which evolutionary processes have worked so dramatically. The increasing complexity

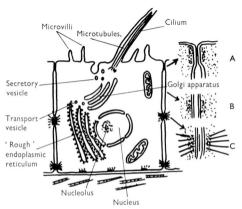

Fig. 5.—Diagrammatic representation of an epithelial cell as seen with the electron microscope. A, B, and C show higher detail of the zonula occludens, zonula adhaerens, and macula adhaerens (desmosome).

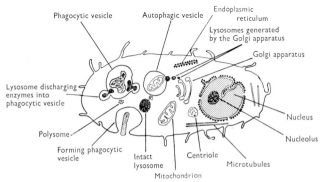

Fig. 6.—Diagram of cell showing components as they might appear under the electron microscope.

of the multicellular organisms is still dependent upon the collective functioning of individual cells, each of which displays features common to all other cells in addition to features specific to its cell type.

All cells contain certain components of distinctive size and shape, having a characteristic structure when viewed in the electron microscope and each contributing individually or collectively to the normal functioning of that cell; these components are termed 'organelles'. Most of the basic components of a cell are represented diagrammatically in *Figs.* 5 and 6. On the basis of electron microscopical studies, all organelles seen with the light microscope are now known to be formed on a skeleton of unit membranes. The membranous structures include the cell membrane, mitochondria, Golgi apparatus, and endoplasmic reticulum, all of which have the same basic physical structure. Membrane components separate compartments such as the outside of the cell from the inside, or the contents of a vesicle from the cytoplasm; they also act as a surface for enzyme action, especially in mitochondria.

MEMBRANES

Structurally, unit membranes are generally considered to consist largely of a double chain of phospholipid molecules, each having a hydrophilic and a hydrophobic end. The hydrophilic groups line up along the outer

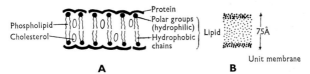

A   B

Fig. 7.—A, Diagram of structure of plasma membrane. B, Image of plasma membrane as seen in electron microscope section.

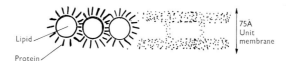

Fig. 8.—Diagram illustrating the newer 'globular' theory of unit membrane structure.

surfaces of the double membrane and are bound, together with other lipid molecules, to proteins. The hydrophobic ends form the inside of the sandwich (*Fig.* 7). Although such a membrane is only 70–100 Å thick, it appears in electron micrographs of fixed cells as a distinct double line, which it is thought is due to the interaction between the fixative used and the protein and polar groups. Recently, this concept of membrane organization has been challenged and there is now strong evidence that the lipid component is in the form of a globule with the protein surrounding each globule (*Fig.* 8). Whatever the exact organization of the unit membrane, it is such that there can be a wide variation in the composition of the lipid and great diversity of the protein, especially the enzymes, without changing the fundamental function of the membrane, that of separating two environments.

The Cell Membrane.—Each cell is surrounded by a cell membrane which forms a selective physical barrier between the cytoplasm and the extracellular compartment. Animal cell surfaces are nearly always irregular in shape with projections ranging in size from the large pseudopodia extending from some mobile cells, to the very much smaller, specialized, finger-like microvilli and cilia of some epithelial cells (*Fig.* 5). In addition the cell membrane may be invaginated to form pinocytotic vesicles containing fluid withdrawn from outside the cell, or phagocytic vesicles for the ingestion of more solid material (*Fig.* 6). Later in this chapter, when considering secretory cells and their functioning, it will be shown that substances produced within the cell often come to be contained within membranous vesicles which move to the cell periphery there to discharge their contents into the extracellular compartment by a process known as 'reverse pinocytosis'. An exception is the collagen macromolecule. How this is secreted by the fibroblast is not known (*see* Chapter IX).

Contact between Cells.—Many cells, particularly epithelial cells, have specialized areas of the cell membrane by which they establish and maintain close contact with their neighbours. Three types of contact structures are recognized from electron micrographs, viz., terminal bars (tight junctions or zonulae occludens), intermediate junctions (zonulae adhaerens), and desmosomes (maculae adhaerens).

Terminal bars are sited between cells towards their end furthest away from the basement membrane; here the electron-dense outer zones of adjacent cell membranes fuse and obliterate the intercellular space to form a continuous belt-like attachment. A band of electron-dense cytoplasm is found associated with this junction (*Fig.* 5A). Intermediate junctions are found between the cells midway along their length where the neighbouring cell membranes are strictly parallel for a short distance though separated by some homogeneous, amorphous material of low density; there are conspicuous bands of dense material in the subjacent cytoplasm (*Fig.* 5B). Desmosomes are present between cells proximal to the basement membrane at points where neighbouring cell membranes separate to generate a localized intercellular space approximately 240 Å wide. This space is filled with a button-like condensation of electron-dense material. Tonofibrils radiate out into the cytoplasm from associated areas of dense material (*Fig.* 5C).

Cell adhesion is particularly important in the gut, for example, where the contents of the gut lumen are prevented from passing between the cells of the gut wall and mixing with the delicately balanced tissue fluids. Similar specialized contact areas found between the ameloblasts are thought to maintain cell cohesion against the forces generated by intrinsic folding of the layer during growth of the tooth germ (*see* Chapter VII).

THE NUCLEUS

Owing to the great affinity of the nucleus for histological stains it quickly became recognized as a component of all viable cells. Moreover, with improvements in the optical microscope and in staining techniques, coupled with the appreciation of its vital role in cell multiplication, the nucleus became almost the sole centre of cytological investigations for many years, the cytoplasm being largely neglected. The chromatin content of the nucleus and its relationship to the maintenance of cell lineage was quickly appreciated, but the precise mechanisms at work remained purely speculative until recent years. It then became known that the primary chemical substance of the genes was deoxyribonucleic acid (DNA), and furthermore that very large molecules composed of this DNA were responsible for carrying the specific information that enabled the cell to express its individuality. We now know that, apart from mitochondrial DNA and certain types of cells which appear to have small quantities in their cytoplasm, DNA is entirely located within the nucleus.

The nucleus of the cell is bounded by a double unit membrane containing numerous pores through which the contents of the nucleus are in contact with the cytoplasm. Within the nucleus are the chromosomes, which consist of very long double chains of DNA. Each long chain is subdivided into smaller units, the genes. The DNA is the master plan, in the form of templates, of all the activities of the body at the cellular level and every cell of one individual contains precisely the same set of templates. Current theory indicates that the functional state of a cell is the result of the activity of the DNA of that cell. For example, a part of the genetic information contained in the DNA may become permanently blocked and therefore rendered ineffective and this represents a permanent change in that cell, in other words the cell has differentiated. Alternatively, parts of the DNA chain may be selectively activated or suppressed, depending on the functional requirements of the cell, and this change is a reversible one. Therefore, in terms of function, cells differ solely in which parts of the plans they use. Thus a fibroblast can be distinguished because it makes use of those parts of the DNA chain which contain the plans for collagen formation, an ameloblast those parts concerned with enamel matrix formation. However, the master plans (DNA) remain almost exclusively within the nucleus and only copies of the relevant parts of them are carried into the cytoplasm by means of a form of ribonucleic acid known as 'messenger' ribonucleic acid ('messenger' RNA), which is manufactured on the templates of the DNA in the nucleus.

Experimental procedures involving the injection of radioactive inorganic phosphate into animal tissues, whereby the RNA molecule is labelled, show the initial labelling only in the nucleolus. Only with the passing of time is there labelling of the cytoplasmic RNA. These and similar results strongly suggest that RNA is only synthesized in the nucleus, whence the molecules migrate into the cytoplasm. 'Messenger' RNA may thus be regarded as the co-ordinating agent between nucleus and cytoplasm. More refined techniques suggest, however, that there may also be some RNA synthesis in the cytoplasm, but as yet the evidence is rather inconclusive.

The relationship between nucleus and cytoplasm has been elegantly demonstrated by removing the nuclei from single-celled animals, (protozoa). These experiments show that the cell is only capable of performing all its functions when nucleus and cytoplasm are in mutual coexistence.

The above account leads to the conclusion that the function of the nucleus is twofold. It contains the DNA which is responsible for the maintenance of cell lineage, although it must be remembered that recognizable chromosomes containing the DNA are only visible during mitosis. This same DNA is in reality the coded information which, during the life span of the cell, is passed to those centres of the cytoplasm whose function is to control the synthesis and release of selected proteins required at any one moment.

PROTEIN SYNTHESIS

Under the light microscope the cytoplasm of the living cell appears to consist of a clear, colourless material within which countless opaque particles are in constant random movement. The electron microscope reveals even more structures (organelles) within the cytoplasm of the fixed cell. In many cells the organelles for protein synthesis are prominent; these consist of ribosomes composed of a second form of RNA and the associated endoplasmic reticulum (*see below*). It will be recalled that 'messenger' RNA is synthesized within the nucleus on the templates of DNA. From here, the 'messenger' RNA carries its information, also in the form of templates, to cytoplasmic aggregations of 'ribosomal' RNA where protein is synthesized by joining together amino-acids.

The bonds connecting amino-acids in a polypeptide chain do not form spontaneously, for when amino-acids are mixed in a test-tube no linkage occurs. For linkage to occur energy is required. Energy in the form of adenosine triphosphate (ATP) is donated enzymatically within the cell and the amino-acid is spoken of as being 'activated'. The activated amino-acid is brought to the ribosome by one of a series of 'transfer' or soluble RNA molecules (the third form of RNA) each of which is specific for a particular amino-acid. In the ribosome the 'transfer' RNA molecules, with their attached activated amino-acids, take their appropriate places on the template so that the amino-acids are alined and held in proper sequence to form a specific polypeptide chain. The complex of 'ribosomal' 'messenger' RNA, and 'transfer' RNA, plus the forming polypeptide chain, together constitute the polysome. A good analogy here is the automated machine tool. The ribosome represents the machine tool, the 'messenger' RNA the tape with its coded instructions, and the 'transfer' RNA is the conveyor belt bringing the raw materials.

Endoplasmic Reticulum and Golgi Apparatus.—It appears that there are two main paths of protein production: one for the replacement of cell components or for retention within the cell, the other for the synthesis of protein for secretion from the cell. Protein for internal use is produced by ribosomes distributed within the cytoplasm most frequently in groups forming 'rosettes' (*Fig.* 6). Cells which undergo keratinization are of this type, having evenly distributed 'rosettes', a simple and relatively insignificant Golgi apparatus, and a demonstrably increasing number of retained protein filaments in their cytoplasm (*Fig.* 9). In cells such as mucous cells and ameloblasts where proteins are produced for secretion the mechanism is slightly different. Here the ribosomes are associated with the surface of the endoplasmic reticulum which is composed of a series of flattened interconnected vesicles, giving the reticulum a 'rough' appearance in electron micrographs (*Fig.* 5). The protein synthesized on the ribosomes passes into the lumen of this 'rough' endoplasmic reticulum and may be secreted directly from there.

More commonly the products pass from the 'rough' endoplasmic reticulum into the lumen of the 'smooth' endoplasmic reticulum (so called on account of the absence of associated ribosomes) or Golgi apparatus (*Fig.* 5). As more and more of the secretory material accumulates the 'smooth' endoplasmic reticulum swells and buds off to form discrete secretory vesicles. In the pancreas, for example, the secretory vesicles contain the pancreatic enzymes, or in goblet cells the secretion is mucus. Gradually the secretory vesicles move to the free border of the cell where

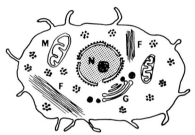

Fig. 9.—Diagram of a protein-retaining cell. Note the poorly formed Golgi apparatus (G), evenly scattered 'rosettes', and absence of rough membranes. F, Retained protein fibres; M, Mitochondrion; N, Nucleolus in the nucleus.

their encompassing membrane fuses with the cell membrane, a break appears in the cell surface and the contents of the vesicle are extruded from the cell by a secretory vesicle (*Fig.* 5). Recent work has shown that the Golgi apparatus is not just a series of passively distensible sacs but that it can modify the proteins passing through by attaching carbohydrates to them.

Lysosomes.—The Golgi apparatus is also concerned with the production of lysosomes. These cytoplasmic bodies (*Fig.* 6) are concentrations of active hydrolytic enzymes surrounded by a single membrane. There are more than twenty lysosomal enzymes and they are all active at an acid pH. Lysosomal enzymes are found in the Golgi apparatus and lysosomes are formed by the pinching off of small vesicles from the edges of the Golgi saccules (*Fig.* 6). When a human macrophage or a phagocytic animal like an amoeba ingests solid material, tissue debris, or an organism, a phagocytic vesicle is formed (*Fig.* 6). Cytoplasmic lysosomes fuse with this vesicle, their enzymes are discharged into it, and the contained phagocytosed material is broken down.

In addition to the breakdown of material in phagocytic vesicles, lysosomal enzymes are employed to break down damaged or unwanted organelles like mitochondria. This takes place in 'autophagic' vesicles. The organelle is first isolated from the cytoplasm by a membrane thereby forming a vesicle into which lysosomal enzymes are injected. In this way the cell is able selectively to eliminate single organelles without digesting other cytoplasmic components.

MITOCHONDRIA AND ENERGY PRODUCTION

Processes such as protein synthesis and other functions performed by cells require energy. This energy is mainly derived from the breakdown of high-energy phosphate compounds such as adenosine triphosphate (ATP); mitochondria are the main source of ATP production. The cytoplasm of all living cells, except bacteria and mature red blood-cells, contains numerous mitochondria. They may vary considerably in outline but all have an outer limiting membrane within which there is an additional membrane, infolded to produce a pattern of cristae that serve to increase the surface area of the interior for catalytic purposes. Most recent work shows that mitochondria divide and grow, rather than arising *de novo*, or from non-mitochondral precursors.

Highly refined biochemical techniques have shown that the mitochondria contain numerous enzymes. Some of these enzymes are concerned with the Krebs cycle. This involves the progressive oxidation of a succession of organic acids, each stage being governed by a different and specific enzyme. At various parts of the cycle energy is generated and CO_2 released. This is a true cycle in that the starting substrate is reconstituted at the end and is ready to re-run the cycle provided the requisite enzyme is available. Much of the energy produced in the mitochondria is used to reconstitute ATP. This substance is used in various processes in many parts of the cell, for when it is broken down it releases the energy again. The mitochondria may thus be regarded as centres of energy production within the cell, in fact they are the 'power house' of the cell.

MICROTUBULES

A group of intracellular structures whose importance has only recently been recognized is the microtubular system. These microtubules (*Figs.* 5, 6) may be several micra in length, typically 250 Å in diameter, and have an electron dense wall which under the highest powers of magnification contains a number of filamentous units, the central core being appreciably less electron dense, though it is doubtful whether it is patent. The tubules show no evidence of branching, are remarkably straight and available evidence shows them to be stiff and elastic with a high tendency to return to the straight form after distortion. Microtubules appear to perform three main functions. First, they arise from the centrioles during cell division and provide the spindle along which the chromosomes separate. Second, sheaths of the tubules form the motile element of cilia and flagella and, third, microtubules appear to play a role in the transport of substances through cytoplasm though this function has not yet been conclusively demonstrated. In connexion with the latter function it is significant that they are particularly prominent in cells with long processes such as odontoblasts and neurons where the extremities of the cell may be a very long way from the nuclear region.

We have so far described the structure and functioning of the cell in isolation, but in the multicellular animal relatively few cells exist in isolation. The multicellular grade of organization confers upon an animal a great variety of advantages over its unicellular ancestor not the least of which is the great potential for evolutionary changes developing in such cellular agglomerations. The setting aside of certain groups of cells, some to perform one and some another function for the good of the entire animal, is the process by which tissues and organs evolve. These are but steps in the process of cell and tissue differentiation and the establishment of the division of labour within the multicellular organism.

We have seen that, apart from viruses, the cell forms the fundamental unit of all living matter and whatever their ultimate function all cells are but modifications of a basic type. We have briefly touched upon the concept of the tissue and of the organ, wherein intercellular co-operation permits functional specialization and division of labour, the advent of which is recognized as being a step of fundamental importance in the evolution of progressive forms of animal life. Within the remaining chapters of this book the concept of functional specialization of the cell will be extended and developed in so far as it is concerned with the production of the definitive human tooth.

REFERENCES

BUTLER, J. A. V. (1959), *Inside the Living Cell*. London: Allen & Unwin.

CHEDD, G. (1968), 'Ribosomes: The Assembly Shops of Life—1', *New Scient.*, **39**, No. 607, 175.

— — (1968), 'Ribosomes: The Assembly Shops of Life—2', *Ibid.*, **39**, No. 608, 233.

FARQUHAR, M. G., and PALADE, G. E. (1963), 'Junctional Complexes in Various Epithelia', *J. cell Biol.*, **17**, 375.

JACOB, F., and MONOD, J. (1961), 'Genetic Regulatory Mechanisms in the Synthesis of Proteins', *J. mol. Biol.*, **3**, 318.

The Living Cell (1965), Readings from *Scientific American*. With Introduction by Donald Kennedy. San Francisco: Freeman.

LOEWY, A. G., and SIEKEVITZ, R. (1963), *Cell Structure and Function*. London: Holt, Rinehart & Winston.

MERCER, E. H. (1963), *Cells and Cell Structure*. London: Hutchinson.

NEUTRA, M., and LEBLOND, C. P. (1969), 'The Golgi Apparatus', *Scient. Am.*, **220**, 100.

PORTER, K. R. (1966), 'Cytoplasmic Microtubules and their Functions', in *Principles of Bimolecular Organization* (ed. WOLSTENHOLME, G. E. W., and O'CONNOR, M.). London: Churchill.

REITH, E. J. (1968), 'Ultrastructural Aspects of Dentinogenesis', in *Dentine and Pulp: Their Structure and Reactions* (ed. SYMONS, N. B. B.). London: Livingstone.

CHAPTER III

THE TOOTH IN SITU

THIS brief description of the developing and completed human tooth in situ is meant to introduce the student to the terminology and position of the salient tissues as they might appear in a section of a human jaw. The composite diagrams in *Figs.* 10 and 11 are meant to provide a glossary of components rather than an accurate histological picture. The boxed numbers appearing alongside some of the structures and tissues labelled in *Fig.* 11 refer to the chapter in this book dealing specifically with the features in question, so that the diagrams may also serve as a rapid index.

The forming tooth germ (*Fig.* 10) has reached the bell stage of development, during which tissues concerned with crown production are rapidly differentiating.

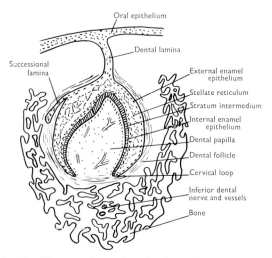

Fig. 10.—Diagram of a section of a developing tooth in situ.

The enamel organ comprises an outer enamel epithelium which is continuous with the basal layer of the oral epithelium via the dental lamina. At the cervical loop, the outer enamel epithelium folds sharply and continues over the surface of the papilla as the inner enamel epithelium. Adjacent to the inner enamel epithelium, and within the enamel organ, is a layer of stratified cells forming the stratum intermedium. The enamel organ is occupied by a diffuse stellate reticulum which is largely composed of intercellular fluid-filled spaces.

The richly vascular dental papilla contains the many types of cells found in any connective tissue. Its surface is lined by odontoblasts whose chief function is to produce dentine.

Each tooth germ is separated from the alveolar bone by its own fibrous tooth follicle which expands as the tooth grows.

On the lingual side of the tooth germ, in the region of its attachment to the dental lamina, a successional lamina develops at whose deep edge grows the germ of the permanent tooth.

The nerve and vascular supplies to the tooth germ are derived from main trunks lying beneath its base.

The completed and functional tooth (*Fig.* 11) consists of an enamel covered anatomical crown and a cement-covered anatomical root. The term 'anatomical crown' must be distinguished from the term 'clinical

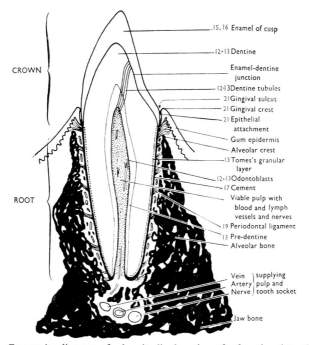

Fig. 11.—Composite diagram of a longitudinal section of a functional tooth in situ.

crown'. The clinical crown is that part of the tooth which is exposed in the mouth at any given age. In young persons part of the base of the anatomical crown remains hidden by the gingival margin so that the clinical crown is smaller than the anatomical crown. In elderly persons the gingival margin retreats rootwards (passive eruption), exposing the entire anatomical crown and also often a small portion of the anatomical root. The clinical crown is now larger than the anatomical crown.

The anatomical root is all that part of the tooth lying deep to the level of the cervical margin of the enamel and typically contained within the bony alveolus (socket). Enamel is not normally present on the root except as enamel droplets, commonly found in the root bifurcations of molars.

By far the greatest proportion of a tooth consists of dentine, a mineralized tissue permeated throughout its thickness by regularly arranged dentine tubules, each containing a fine protoplasmic process of an odontoblast cell which is itself situated on the surface of the pulp. The outer surface of the coronal dentine lines the enamel-dentine junction which is microscopically irregular. A further mineralized tissue, cement, lies on the outer surface of the root and serves as an attachment for fibres of the periodontal ligament (*see below*). Immediately beneath the surface of the root dentine there is a microscopically granular layer, termed the 'granular layer of Tomes'. In the centre of the coronal dentine is the pulp chamber which in a young tooth extends as a pulp horn beneath the cusp. A pulp canal runs the entire length of each root and opens into the periodontal ligament at the apical foramen. The tissue within the pulp cavity is a normal connective tissue covered by specialized cells, the odontoblasts.

Enamel is the refractile microcrystalline, highly mineralized layer on the outer surface of the anatomical crown.

The only site where oral epithelium comes into direct contact with the functional tooth is at the base of the clinical crown. Here the epithelium is turned inwards and attached to the surface of the enamel, producing the gingival sulcus and the epithelial attachment.

The tooth is anchored to its socket in the alveolar bone by the collagen fibres of the periodontal ligament. Most of these fibres run obliquely and coronally from the cement into the alveolar bone. The bundles of fibres which are inserted into the mineralized tissues are called 'Sharpey's fibres'. The term 'alveolar bone' refers to that part of the jaw which contains holes (alveoli). It is not in any way histologically distinguishable from the remaining bone tissue of the jaws. It exists solely to support the teeth and is largely resorbed when the teeth are lost.

CHAPTER IV

THE ROLE OF ECTOMESENCHYME IN TOOTH FORMATION

THE neural crest is an important and complex primordium found in the early embryo. The fertilized egg rapidly develops to form an embryonic disk consisting of two cell types, an outer layer of ectoderm and an inner layer of endoderm. The space between these two germ layers comes to be occupied by a third germ layer, the mesoderm, thus establishing the triploblastic embryo. At this time the longitudinal axis of the embryo is emphasized by the formation of the neural plate as a symmetrical demarcated area of ectoderm, wider at the future head end, bounded by thickened marginal folds, and extending along the future dorsal surface (*Fig.* 12).

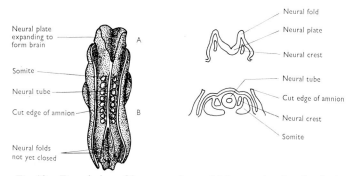

Fig. 12.—Dorsal view of human embryo of 2·1 mm. showing developing central nervous system. To the right, diagrammatic cross-sections at levels A and B.

In time, the neural folds rise up and, approaching each other, meet and fuse along the midline, thus converting the neural plate into a tube which sinks inwards beneath the surface ectoderm. During the development of the neural tube small groups of ectodermal cells break away from the margins of the neural plate and come to lie parallel to, and on either side of, the neural tube. These constitute the neural crest cells. The mesoderm gives rise to mesenchyme (mesodermal mesenchyme) from which differentiate a wide range of cells and tissues such as fibrous tissue, adipose tissue, tendons, and ligaments. The neural crest is the source of a tremendous variety of cell and tissue types: pigment cells, Schwann cells, the meninges of the brain, the cells of the spinal and autonomic ganglia, the adrenal medulla, large amounts of mesenchyme (called either 'mesectoderm' or 'ectomesenchyme') from some of which, by further induction, the branchial arch cartilages and the dental papillae of developing teeth differentiate.

The refined techniques of experimental embryology have extended our knowledge of the role of neural crest far beyond the limitations associated with the examination of serial sections of normal embryos. Much of this work, involving delicate ablation, extirpation, and transplantation of neural crest tissue, has been performed on larval forms of fish and amphibia and also on chick embryos. In some of these animals the ectomesenchymal cells are pigmented and free of yolk, differing from the yolk-laden surrounding mesenchymal cells. This enables them to be traced for some time in sections of the embryos. Marking such cells with intra-vitam dyes, or more recently with radioactively labelled compounds, greatly eases the following of their migratory routes during development.

The collective information obtained from these experiments shows without doubt that, in the early developing stages of these vertebrates, the branchial arch cartilages from which the jaws arise are formed from ectomesenchyme which has migrated downwards from near the mid-dorsal line. Moreover, while the formation of the mouth depends upon the inductive interaction between ectoderm and endoderm, no teeth develop in jaws unless ectomesenchyme is also present. De Beer (1947) was able to show conclusively that the odontoblasts of larval salamander teeth were of ectomesenchymal origin, and that in this animal some of the enamel organs were of ectodermal and others of endodermal origin. Hence, he concludes that the ectomesenchyme is the primary factor in inducing the formation of the enamel organ from the overlying surface epithelium irrespective of its origin.

Experiments on mammalian embryos comparable with those on amphibian larvae are not possible. However, such observations as it has been possible to make on mammals lend support to the view that in general the findings in amphibians can be cautiously applied to mammals. It is well established that in very early embryos areas of morphogenesis tend to be rich in RNA, and that gradients of RNA concentration signify gradients of morphogenetic or metabolic activity. Furthermore, the distribution of alkaline phosphatase, one of whose associations is with protein synthesis, is very similar to that of RNA and also such areas of high metabolic activity are often transiently rich in glycogen. These properties have been used to observe in the mouse bands of ectomesenchyme streaming into the maxillary and mandibular processes (*Fig.* 13) there to congregate beneath the surface ectoderm, at a time before the latter shows any evidence of the thickening which is generally recognized as the initial stage of the process which will lead to tooth formation.

It is now widely recognized that in addition to having high concentrations of RNA, alkaline phosphatase, and glycogen, regions of intense morphogenesis are also the sites of blood vascular concentration. In the embryo cat, which has been closely studied, the capillary vascular system within the mesenchyme underlying the future position of the tooth germs is established before there is any evidence of epithelial thickening. Even at a slightly later stage, an increase in the capillary density occurs in relation to the dental lamina at the sites of future tooth germs, before corresponding epithelial activity. Hence, it is possible to predict the location of the tooth buds and of diastemata by observing the distribution of capillary density along the length of the jaw.

It must be apparent to the reader that none of these observations is related specifically to the human embryo. However, it is reasonable to suppose that the embryo mouse or cat is not radically different from the human embryo.

From the above evidence it is clear that ectomesenchyme plays an important role in the organization of the tissues of the vertebrate jaws, including the teeth. However, it would be unwise to state that the ecto-mesenchyme solely induces the development of the ectodermal component of the tooth. During the past few years a great deal of work has been done with tissue culture techniques on epithelial-mesenchymal interactions by separating them with an inert membrane specially manufactured for such studies. With this technique epithelium and mesenchyme are first separated and then *in vitro* brought together on either side of the inert membrane.

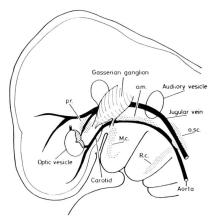

Fig. 13.—Diagram showing the distribution of mesenchyme rich in alkaline phosphatase (stippled) in the head region of a 10-day mouse embryo. Vessels supplying the branchial arches are omitted. M.c., precursor of Meckel's cartilage; o.m., primordium of external rectus muscle; o.sc., occipital sclerotomes; pr., premandibular area; R.c., precursor of Reichert's cartilage. (*Reproduced from Milaire, J.*, 1959, *Archs Biol., Liège*, **70**, 587.)

Using this technique, mesenchyme from different sources can be brought close to epithelia taken from different sites in the body and the effects of one on the other studied. Certain general principals have emerged. The epithelium is dependent upon the presence of mesenchyme or a factor produced by the mesenchyme for its continued development. The epithelium is specific. For example, presumptive pancreatic epithelium associated with salivary gland mesenchyme differentiates into pancreatic gland cells. In addition to its generalized inductive effect mesenchyme also has a specific effect. Thus salivary mesenchyme with salivary epithelium gives rise to glandular salivary epithelium whereas salivary epithelium with jaw mesenchyme results in the maintenance of the epithelium but glandular cells are not differentiated. Indeed, it now seems most likely that embryonic induction involves a two-way interaction. Not only does the mesenchyme induce epithelium, but the epithelium also acts back on the mesenchyme.

REFERENCES

DE BEER, G. R. (1947), 'The Differentiation of Neural Crest Cells into Visceral Cartilages and Odontoblasts in *Ambystoma*, and a Re-examination of the Germ-layer Theory', *Proc. R. Soc.*, **B-134**, 377.

FLEISCHMAJER, R., and BILLINGHAM, R. E. (1968), *Epithelial-Mesenchymal Interactions*. Baltimore: Williams & Wilkins.

GAUNT, W. A. (1959), 'The Vascular Supply to the Dental Lamina during Early Development', *Acta anat.*, **37**, 232.

— — and MILES, A. E. W. (1967), 'Fundamental Aspects of Tooth Morphogenesis', in *Structural and Chemical Organization of Teeth* (ed. MILES, A. E. W.), vol. 1. New York: Academic.

HÖRSTADIUS, S. (1950), *The Neural Crest*. London: Oxford University Press.

Chapter V

THE EARLY DEVELOPMENT OF THE TEETH

It is not intended to give here a detailed account of the histological changes which have been observed during development of the human tooth. The reader is referred to standard texts for complete details.

The epithelium in the front of the definitive mouth is derived from the lining of the original invaginated stomatodeum and is accordingly of ectodermal origin. Further back in the mouth the oral lining is derived from the endoderm of the embryonic pharynx, though the precise line of demarcation is a point of controversy (*Fig.* 14). Certainly, there is no detectable histological distinction to be seen in tissue sections taken through regions where the bucco-pharyngeal membrane has broken down

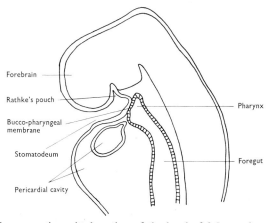

Fig. 14.—Diagrammatic sagittal section of the head of 2·5-mm. human embryo. Tissue of endodermal origin is cross-hatched.

At the time of initiation of the processes which will result in tooth formation, the potential tooth-bearing areas and the lips are covered by a considerably thicker layer of epithelial cells than the remainder of the primitive pharynx. These cells are rich in glycogen but, because glycogen is lost in the normal preparation of tissues for histological sectioning, the cells may appear vacuolated.

Studies of closely timed series of mouse embryos show that the first indication of the processes which will result in tooth formation consists of a condensation of ectomesenchyme tissue immediately beneath the surface epithelium, along the tooth-bearing region of each jaw (*Fig.* 15A). The condensation first appears at the front of the mouth, close to the midline, and spreads steadily backwards along each jaw quadrant, that in the lower jaw being slightly in advance of the upper. The precocity of the developmental processes in the lower jaw persists throughout ontogeny. This condensation of ectomesenchyme is probably responsible for the primary inductive influence in tooth formation referred to in the previous chapter. However, blood-capillaries are more numerous in the region of the ectomesenchymal condensation than in other regions of the jaws.

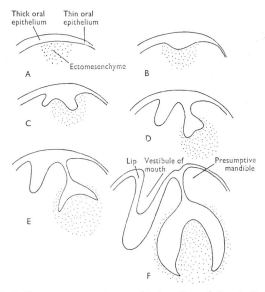

Fig. 15.—Each diagram represents a sagittal section of the skull through the subsequent incisor region.
A, Ectomesenchyme is concentrated beneath the thick pharyngeal epithelium which covers the subsequent tooth bearing region of the jaw. The lip will be to the left. B, The formation of the primary epithelial band. C, The vestibular band pushes anteriorly into the adjacent mesenchyme while the dental lamina grows into the ectomesenchyme. D, A tooth bud forms at the end of the dental lamina. The vestibular band increases in size. E, The ectodermal part of the tooth bud extends around the growing ball of ectomesenchymal cells to produce a cap. F, Continued growth of the ectodermal cells around the growing ball of ectomesenchymal cells results in a bell-shaped enamel organ. The central cells of the vestibular band break down separating a lip on the left from the subsequent alveolar region of the jaw on the right.

Following closely on this the oral epithelium adjacent to the ectomesenchyme begins to proliferate and protrudes into the underlying cellular condensation (*Fig.* 15B). The epithelial prominence is referred to as the 'primary epithelial band'. The position of the primary epithelial band may be controlled by a prior genetic determination of either the position at which the ectomesenchyme condenses, or by the sprouting of capillary networks, or by both. Frequent references are made in textbooks of embryology to the unbroken continuity of the primary epithelial band across the midline of the developing mammalian jaw. However, recent work shows quite clearly that in mouse, cat, and human embryos the band develops individually in each jaw quadrant, only uniting in the midline anteriorly in the 15 mm. C.R. stage human embryo.

At this stage the primary epithelial band is shaped like a horseshoe (more accurately, a catenary), following the outline of the subsequent dental arcade. While continuing to proliferate into the ectomesenchyme the primary epithelial band starts pushing a buccal extension into the adjacent mesenchyme (*Fig.* 15C). The former extension is now referred to as the 'dental lamina' and the buccal extension as the 'vestibular lamina'.

Standard textbook descriptions imply that the dental lamina progressively invades the underlying ectomesenchyme so that as individual tooth germs bud from it they progressively come to lie deeper within the jaw. However, an alternative explanation seems possible. Namely, that on each side of the dental lamina the ectomesenchymal cells proliferate and push the oral epithelium towards the cavity of the pharynx away from the developing tooth germs, stretching the connexion (the dental lamina) between them. When, in later developmental stages, the lamina breaks down, severing this connexion, it appears to be split apart in tissue sections, an appearance which accords well with the above suggestion.

The ectomesenchymal cells adjacent to the growing end of the dental lamina now appear to clump in regions which correspond with those of the subsequent tooth germs. Just as in the earlier stages of tooth development when the whole dental lamina proliferated into the ectomesenchyme, so at this later stage, following the regional clumping of ectomesenchyme, stalks of dental lamina continue proliferating into the now localized condensations. These stalks and the adjacent ectomesenchyme are the tooth buds (*Fig.* 15D).

The above account of the differentiation of the earliest tooth buds is the one most usually given. However, there is an alternative interpretation of the microscopical appearances seen in tissue sections of these very early human embryos. This suggests that the ectodermal parts of the deciduous incisors, canines, and first deciduous molars actually develop within the primary epithelial band rather than in the later formed dental lamina. The reason for this difference is that it is very difficult to be certain of when a group of ectodermal cells has clumped together to form the *anlage* of an enamel organ. Some workers consider that they have evidence that the cells of the presumptive enamel organs can be seen to be clumped together before the primary epithelial band has divided into a vestibular and dental lamina.

The ectomesenchymal cells continue to proliferate thereby increasing the size of the ball of cells adjacent to the epithelial part of the tooth bud. But the epithelium itself continues to proliferate in what might be described as an attempt to surround the growing ball of ectomesenchymal cells. Some of the ectomesenchymal cells become pushed aside and are to be found around the edges of the encircling epithelial cells. The encircling attempts are 'more successful' and the epithelium spreads out to form a cap of cells on top of the ectomesenchyme (*Fig.* 15E). This is the cap stage of tooth development. It is during this stage that histo-differentiation begins, the definitive tissues of the dental organ differentiating, each to play a specific role in the generation of the completed tooth. As the epithelial cap grows, its central cells become increasingly separated from the vascular ectomesenchyme. The innermost cells begin to secrete acidic mucopolysaccharides into the narrow intercellular spaces separating them (*Fig.* 16). The mucopolysaccharides are intensely hydrophilic and water is pulled into the intercellular spaces, compressing the cytoplasm of each of the cells within the inner mass. All the cells of the enamel organ are united by desmosomes and despite the compression of their cytoplasm the desmosomal connexions between the inner cells are maintained. This process results in the development of a stellate reticulum whose intercellular spaces are filled with water and mucopolysaccharides.

Owing to the appearance of intercellular fluid-filled spaces the stellate reticulum is transformed into a turgid diffuse tissue whose functions may be considered under two headings, mechanical and nutritional. In a mechanical sense, it has been suggested that the stellate reticulum serves

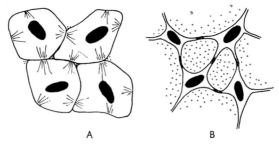

A   B

Fig. 16.—A, Four polygonal cells within the centre of the enamel organ secrete mucopolysaccharides (stippled) into the intercellular region. The mucopolysaccharides are hydrophilic and water is absorbed (B). The desmosomal connexions between the cells are maintained producing the stellate reticulum.

to protect the developing tooth germ against mechanical disturbance from without, and also to provide the requisite space for crown development within the tooth follicle. It has also been suggested that the tissue's turgor pressure serves to maintain the spherical shape of the dental organ during development and at the same time to balance the growth pressures generated by the expanding dental papilla (ectomesenchyme).

Early workers believed that the stellate reticulum provided a source of inorganic salts or ions to be drawn upon enamel formation. However, neither histochemical nor micro-incineration techniques have revealed an abnormally high calcium content in the stellate reticulum either before or during the phase of enamel formation. The stellate reticulum is, however, rich in acidic mucopolysaccharide which generally diminishes during enamel formation. The provision of this substance may well be its main nutritive role.

The epithelial cells adjacent to the ectomesenchyme become cuboidal and then low columnar in shape, the layer being now called the inner enamel epithelium. The cells of the outer enamel epithelium remain roughly cuboidal.

At this time the centre of the inner enamel epithelium is swollen into a mass of cells comprising the enamel knot. Workers in the early part of the nineteenth century attached great importance to this transitory structure believing it acted as a stable 'nucleus' of form-determining function. Closely associated with the knot is a cellular condensation traversing the stellate reticulum to unite with the outer enamel epithelium close to the latter's attachment to the dental lamina. This enamel cord or septum, together with the enamel knot, is now thought to contribute cells to the stellate reticulum.

The outer enamel epithelium plays a passive role in morphogenesis of the crown serving merely to contain the stellate reticulum. It may, however, control the exchange of substances between the enamel organ and its environment. It is continuous with the inner enamel epithelium at the cervical loop where the two epithelia fold sharply upon each other to provide a stable rim to the enamel organ. Much later in time it will be seen that growth of the cervical loop provides the impetus for root formation. In early development the outer enamel epithelium is directly continuous, via the dental lamina, with the oral epithelium: the germ of the successional tooth will develop from its point of union with the lamina. Later the outer enamel epithelium is reinforced by the fibres of the dental follicle to assist in counteracting the internal pressures generated by the growing crown.

The mass of ectomesenchymal cells continues to increase in size but the steady encircling action of the enamel organ also continues until it surrounds such a large part of the dental papilla that the tooth germ takes on the appearance of a bell—the bell stage of tooth development (*Fig.* 15F). It is during this stage that the major cusps, ridges, and fissures of the ultimate crown pattern are established by the folding of the inner enamel epithelium. The dynamics of the folding process will form the subject of the next chapter and no more will be said at this stage.

At the early bell stage of development a new layer of cells differentiates within the enamel organ. This is the stratum intermedium. Presumably this layer is derived from the cells inside the enamel organ, perhaps from the diminishing enamel knot. It has been suggested that cells from this new layer may insinuate between the now columnar cells of the inner enamel epithelium helping to increase the area of this encircling layer.

During development each tooth germ is contained within a collagenous fibrous follicle largely generated by fibroblasts of mesenchymal origin. However, those layers adjacent to the tooth germ are probably derived from ectomesenchymal cells displaced outwards from the presumptive dental papilla by the growing margin of the cervical loop. This innermost layer is vascular and it lies close upon the surface of the outer enamel epithelium. Beneath the tooth germ it is continuous with the deep surface of the dental papilla, the vessels and nerves supplying the latter passing through it. The outer layer of the follicle lies against the walls of the bony crypt, while above the tooth its fibres merge with those of the deep layer of the oral mucosa. The follicle thus separates the developing tooth from the bony crypt.

The follicles of neighbouring teeth are united by fibrous strands along the length of the jaws, suggesting that the fibrous sheathing serves to maintain the correct spacing of the teeth and prevent possible distortion of the tooth row during elongation of the jaws. Within the follicle the developing tooth is able to undergo slight positional adjustments caused by growth forces generated during crown development. At the same time the fibrous layers of the follicle provide sufficient reinforcement to prevent the distortion of the outer enamel epithelium by forces from within the tooth germ. Though some of the follicle is destroyed when the tooth erupts, it will be seen in a later chapter that this tissue forms the basis of the periodontal ligament which maintains the functional tooth in its bony socket.

The application of highly sophisticated experimental techniques to very early developmental stages of amphibia have shown that the early embryo is differentiated into a mosaic of 'organization fields', each making a specific contribution to the definitive animal under the influence of chemical substances called 'evocators'.

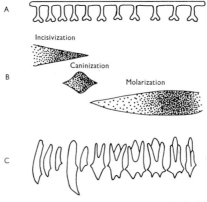

Fig. 17.—Diagrammatic representation of hypothetical differentiation of the mammalian dentition. A, The dental lamina with undifferentiated tooth germs; B, Morphogenetic fields believed to influence the development of the tooth germs; C, The resulting definitive dentition. (*Reproduced from Butler*, 1939.)

In general terms, an anteroposterior (head-tail) polarity is established at an early stage in the developing embryo. The anterior pole is more advanced and from here a gradient of differentiation diminishes towards the posterior region. Within this major gradient further minor gradients develop. The major gradient results in (for instance) the successive differentiation of vertebrae which are probably all built up under the control of the same genetic influence; bodies, pedicles, laminae, and transverse processes are common to all but there is a gradual variation between successive vertebrae. Such a series is known as a 'meristic' series. The dentition may be another meristic series built from a minor gradient. Each tooth is based on a common plan of root, crown, and pulp chamber. Each quadrant of the mammalian dentition is thought to arise within a continuous morphogenetic field or gradient extending throughout the length of the jaw quadrant. Within this minor gradient there are fields of incisivation, caninization, and molarization such that according to which of these morphogenetic influences acts upon it, the undifferentiated tooth germ produces one or other of these tooth forms (*Fig.* 17).

It will be observed that although there is some overlapping of the fields each has its own locus of maximum effect. In the human dentition the first permanent molar is most greatly influenced by the molarization field, the second and third molars to a lesser degree. This hypothesis provides a feasible step in the explanation of such phenomena as, for example, the molarization of the premolars in the dentition of the horse. It suggests that in this animal the molarization field extends as far forwards as the caninization field which is, however, poorly developed. However, it must be stated that there is no evidence to support this theory; it is merely a useful concept.

In this chapter we have discussed some aspects of the developmental processes affecting the tooth germ through its early stages up to the establishment of its 'bell' form. The next chapter will deal with the morphogenetic processes leading to the generation of the crown topography.

REFERENCES

DE BEER, G. R. (1947), 'The Differentiation of Neural Crest Cells into Visceral Cartilages and Odontoblasts in *Ambystoma*, and a Re-examination of the Germ-layer Theory', *Proc. R. Soc.*, **B-134**, 377.

BUTLER, P. M. (1939), '1. Studies of the Mammalian Dentition. Differentiation of the Post-canine Dentition', *Proc. zool. Soc. Lond.*, **B-109**, 1.

— — (1967), 'Dental Merism and Tooth Development', *J. dent. Res.*, **46**, 845.

FITZGERALD, L. R. (1969), 'Mechanisms controlling Morphogenesis in Developing Teeth', *J. dent. Res.*, **48**, 726.

GAUNT, W. A., and MILES, A. E. W. (1967), 'Fundamental Aspects of Tooth Morphogenesis', in *Structural and Chemical Organisation of Teeth* (ed. MILES, A. E. W.), vol. 1. New York: Academic.

OOÉ, T. (1957), 'On the Early Development of Human Dental Lamina', *Okajimas Folia anat. jap.*, **30**, 197.

POURTOIS, M. (1961), '*Contribution a l'étude des bourgeons dentaires chez la Souris.* 1, *Périodes d'induction et de morphodifferenciation*', *Archs Biol. Liège*, **72**, 17.

SCOTT, J. H. (1967), *Dento-facial Growth and Development*. London: Pergamon.

— — and SYMONS, N. B. B. (1964), *Introduction to Dental Anatomy*. London: Livingstone.

SICHER, H. (1962), *Orban's Oral Histology and Embryology*. St. Louis: Mosby.

TONGE, C. H. (1953), 'The Early Development of Teeth', *Proc. R. Soc. Med.*, **46**, 313.

CHAPTER VI

THE DETERMINATION OF CROWN PATTERN

ALL human lower right first molars look alike and are quite different from those of a cat. The many similarities between the teeth of animals comprising each mammalian species and their differences from the teeth of other mammalian species make it quite obvious that the occlusal morphology of a tooth is to a great extent genetically determined. From a detailed study of molar morphology in identical human twins it has been established that the presence and shape of even quite minor cuspules and fissures are probably genetically determined. Were it not for this study it might have been argued that local mechanical differences accounted for all minor variations between teeth. Similar studies have shown that the shape of the shovel-shaped incisor is also genetically determined. But these genetic studies do not reveal the mechanisms operating on the ball of cells comprising a tooth bud inducing it to develop its own unique shape.

The most obvious and consistent differences between the different teeth of the human dentition are their size, occlusal morphology, and the distribution and number of roots. In this chapter we will consider what is known about the way in which the characteristic occlusal morphology of a tooth is developed.

At the cap stage of tooth development there are obvious differences between the sizes of different tooth germs. These differences can presumably be related to either a more rapid or a longer lasting phase of cell division in the larger tooth germs. However, it is only in the bell stage that distinct morphological differences between tooth germs can be recognized. In the previous chapter a concept was discussed which suggests that these differences are brought about under the influence of tooth fields.

This theory has been investigated in the following way. At a critical stage in the embryonic development of rat teeth the oral epithelium in a jaw quadrant was carefully separated from the underlying mesenchyme and replaced in such a way that the molar epithelium covered the incisor region and the incisor epithelium covered the molar region. The jaw quadrant was now cultured *in vitro*. For a short while the teeth continued to develop in the culture medium. Subsequently these teeth rudiments were studied and it appeared that molariform teeth were developing in the incisor region and incisiform teeth were developing in the molar region. This particular study and other studies on amphibia suggest that different regions of the oral epithelium (rather than the underlying ectomesenchyme) are initially responsible for determining the different occlusal morphologies of teeth. However, the gross differences which have been demonstrated do not establish the existence of gradual morphogenetic gradients, only of gross sites of form determination.

It is during the bell stage of tooth development that the ultimate occlusal morphologies of teeth begin to be established in such a way that it is possible to recognize differences between those germs which will develop into incisor, canine, premolar, and molar teeth. The following theory attempts to explain on a mechanistic basis some of the forces which may be generated within the tooth germ and which may bring about these differences.

The occlusal morphology of a tooth is the outcome of two features. The first is the shape of the enamel-dentine junction. But this shape is not exactly the same as that of the occlusal surface of the tooth. Minor variations, particularly in the form of small cuspules and fissures, are

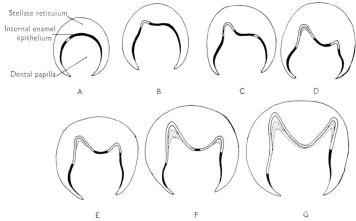

Fig. 18.—Seven stages in the folding of the internal enamel epithelium. Regions in which the cells of the internal enamel epithelium are dividing are black; regions in which division has ceased are clear. Enamel is stippled, dentine is cross-hatched. Cusps continue to separate while the cells of the internal enamel epithelium are dividing. The final shape of the enamel-dentine junction is stabilized when the dentine bridge has connected the two cusps (G).

produced due to regional variations in the thickness of the enamel deposited on the enamel-dentine junction. Apart from documenting their existence no study of the development of these minor variations in enamel thickness appears to have been made, although it has been suggested that the constriction of the blood-supply to ameloblasts in the region of fissures is related to the thin enamel which may be found in these regions. The theory referred to above discusses the way in which the internal enamel epithelium folds to establish the shape of the presumptive enamel-dentine junction. It is only when the first layers of enamel and dentine have been deposited on either side of this junction that its definitive shape is established.

The developing tooth germ may be likened to a fluid-filled sphere which is partitioned across the middle by the inner enamel epithelium. The stellate reticulum is on one side of the partition and the dental papilla on the other side (*Fig.* 18A). The cells of the stellate reticulum are separated from each other by acidic mucopolysaccharide. This substance is intensely hydrophilic and the water which it has absorbed is thought to produce a region of high hydrostatic pressure. On the other side of the partition the growing dental papilla balances this hydrostatic pressure so that the internal enamel epithelium is stabilized between the two. The surrounding dental follicle constricts the tooth germ to an approximately spherical shape. The partitioning sheet of cells (the internal enamel epithelium) increases in surface area by cell division. But its perimeter, the cervical loop, is prevented from expanding by the retaining dental follicle. Evidently, as the surface area of the partition increases it must buckle. By this buckling a primary cuspal elevation of the internal enamel epithelium is produced (*Fig.* 18A, B). From a purely mechanistic analogy it might be thought that the internal enamel epithelium could buckle down

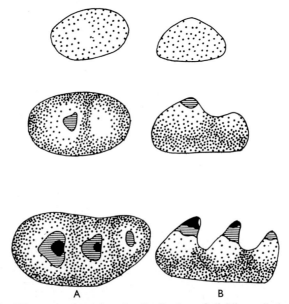

A   B

Fig. 19.—Diagram representing the distribution of dividing cells in the inner dental epithelium of a mouse molar at three successive developmental stages. A, In occlusal view; B, In side view. Not to scale. Solid black area represents forming enamel, lined area forming dentine. Each dot signifies a dividing cell.

into the dental papilla rather than up into the stellate reticulum. But it will be remembered that the surface of the dental papilla is convex towards the internal enamel epithelium and this will result in any mechanical buckling being towards the stellate reticulum.

It has been observed that mitotic activity has now ceased in the region of the cuspal elevation of the internal enamel epithelium and that adjacent odontoblasts rapidly become differentiated and dentine is soon deposited. However, cell division continues in the internal enamel epithelium flanking the primary cuspal elevation. These flanks are now convex towards the dental papilla so that from a purely mechanistic analogy it can be argued that the growing internal enamel epithelium would now begin to buckle into the dental papilla. This does in fact occur so that the height of the primary cuspal elevation is increased by a deepening of its flanks down into the dental papilla rather than further growth up into the stellate reticulum (*Fig.* 18C).

At this stage, if another cusp is to be formed, cell division of the internal enamel epithelium ceases in the region which will correspond with this secondary cusp. Just as in the formation of the primary cusp, so a secondary cuspal elevation develops on the flanks of the now mineralizing primary cusp (*Fig.* 18D). This region becomes rapidly stabilized by the differentiation of odontoblasts and the laying down of dentine. Meanwhile cell division between the two cusps continues so that the internal enamel epithelium buckles further into the papilla thus increasing both the heights and the separation between the now mineralizing cusps (*Fig.* 18E,F,G).

To summarize, it appears that cell division of the sheet of internal enamel epithelium first ceases in the region of what will be the primary cusp of the tooth (*Fig.* 19). This is followed by a buckling of the internal enamel epithelium in this region, the differentiation of odontoblasts, and the laying down of dentine. If further cusps are to be formed cell division in the internal enamel epithelium ceases at the tips of these presumptive secondary cusps which are situated down the flanks of the primary cuspal elevation. The sequence of development of the cusps in equivalent multi-cusped teeth is usually the same.

The cusps of teeth are not the smooth symmetrical cones which would be expected to develop from the simple mechanical explanation given above. Even the human canine possesses ridges running from near the cusp tip to the cervical margin of the crown, while close inspection of unworn molars reveals a variety of ridges associated with each cusp, apparently having little or no functional or phylogenetic significance. While many of these features may be accounted for by localized enamel thickenings, those of a more permanent nature, e.g., the oblique ridges of human upper molars, are established at the enamel dentine junction. Investigation into the distribution of dividing cells in developing molars reveals that growth is not even over the entire surface. Indeed, there is often a greater proportion of dividing cells of the inner enamel epithelium over one flank of a cusp than another, so that it can be argued that tensional forces are set up which cause the cusp to tilt slightly on the crown. This has been shown in the carnassial teeth of the cat. Until mineralization starts the crown pattern remains pliable and ridges can form, to be stabilized later by the formation of hard dentine and enamel along their crests: there is evidence that apposition of enamel spreads more rapidly along the ridges than over the intervening cuspal surfaces. The ridges so formed serve not only to link the cusps and produce a characteristic crown pattern, but also to provide functional shearing edges. Moreover, the complex of ridges tends to generate intervening fossae into which cusps of the opposing teeth can bite to provide a pestle-and-mortar action.

So far little mention has been made regarding the role of the dental papilla in determining the crown pattern. Without the papilla no dentine would form, hence the folds of the inner enamel epithelium would not be stabilized. In fact, early in development the crown pattern is formed in dentine which serves to provide the template over which enamel is later deposited (*Fig.* 18G). In the early stages of development mitosis figures can be observed in the peripheral papilla cells, although the exact correspondence with those in the inner dental epithelium claimed by some does not occur. The papilla follows faithfully the profile of the inner enamel epithelium and may restrain any tendency of the epithelium towards excessive folding. As will become apparent in later chapters, the inner enamel epithelium obtains its nutriment via the papilla until the formation of dentine separates it from this source. Thus the papilla has a nutritive role, at least up to the time of dentine formation. Though there is as yet no direct evidence, it has been argued that growth centres located in the papilla are responsible for controlling the growth in outline of the base of the crown, hence the size of the tooth and incidentally the number and disposition of the roots. Unquestionably the ectodermal and ectomesenchymal components of the tooth germ must work in close co-ordination to produce the topographical pattern of a crown. However, the present state of our knowledge does not allow us to say whether small teeth arise from a small number of initial cells.

It would appear, then, that while the definitive tooth results from developmental interaction between the enamel organ and the dental papilla, the intrinsic growth of the inner enamel epithelium causes this layer to fold in a predetermined manner, so as to generate a genetically reproducible pattern of cusps, ridges, and fissures which become stabilized by the dentine and enamel. In the following chapter we shall review the evidence concerning the role of the soft tissue components of the tooth germ in the context of tooth growth.

REFERENCES

BUTLER, P. M. (1956), 'The Ontogeny of Molar Pattern', *Biol. Rev.*, **31**, 30.

DRYBURG, L. C. (1967), 'The Epigenetics of Early Tooth Development in the Mouse', *J. dent. Res.*, **46**, 1264.

GAUNT, W. A. (1955), 'The Development of the Molar Pattern of the Mouse', *Acta anat.*, **24**, 249.

— — (1959), 'The Development of the Deciduous Cheek Teeth of the Cat', *Ibid.*, **38**, 187.

— — (1961a), 'The Presence of Apical Pits on the Lower Cheek Teeth of the Mouse', *Ibid.*, **44**, 146.

— (1961b), 'The Development of the Molar Pattern of the Golden Hamster', *Ibid.*, **45**, 219.

— — and MILES, A. E. W. (1967), *see* Chapter V.

KRAUS, B. S., and JORDAN, R. E. (1965), *The Human Dentition before Birth*. London: Kimpton.

MILLER, W. A. (1969), 'Inductive Changes in Early Tooth Development: 1, A Study of Mouse Tooth Development on the Chick Chorioallantois', *J. dent. Res.*, **48**, 719.

WOOD, B. F., and GREEN, L. J. (1968), 'Second Premolar Morphologic Trait Similarities in Twins', *Ibid.*, **48**, 74.

CHAPTER VII

GROWTH OF THE TOOTH GERM

THE term 'growth' encompasses all the processes involving increase in size and weight of the individual from the time of fertilization of the egg. In the two preceding chapters some of the histological changes within the tooth germ from its time of inception have been indicated but little has so far been said concerning the progressive changes in the dimensions of the developing tooth germ. In this dimensional sense growth involves changes not only in absolute size but also in the relative proportions of the component parts, both of which determine the definitive form.

Although growth is a progressive and continuous process it seldom proceeds at a constant rate. Characteristically, the life span of the living cell includes a period of high metabolic activity followed by senescence. The cell may now either die or divide. In the latter case there is a renewal of the high metabolic activity. In a dental context, once the cells of the inner enamel epithelium have induced the differentiation of the odontoblasts and have themselves entered upon their secretory phase, their ability to divide is lost. Their remaining contribution to the growth of the crown of the tooth is in the amount of enamel which they are able to secrete before the advent of their senescence.

Before proceeding further it will be helpful to mention briefly some of the techniques available for measuring growth of tooth germs. It is possible by careful microdissection to free the developing tooth germs from the surrounding tissues and to measure their gross dimensions directly. However, owing to the amount of fluid in the stellate reticulum and the delicate nature of the outer enamel epithelium in the early tooth germ, great care is necessary to prevent the enamel organ collapsing and causing distortion of the inner enamel epithelium. With the onset of dentinogenesis, the dentine caps can be dissected out and stained with alizarin red S which differentially stains mineralized regions on the tooth crown. Alternatively, whole jaws may be stained with alizarin red solution and then rendered transparent to allow direct measurements of the stained dentine caps in situ. The total volumes of enamel and dentine formed can be measured directly from dissected teeth. When mineralized the dentine and enamel caps become radio-opaque and their dimensions can be measured directly by radiographs *in vivo*.

However, from the two previous chapters it is clear that much of the crown pattern is defined by the soft tissues before mineralization starts, and that the crown form results from developmental interaction between the enamel organ and the dental papilla, neither of whose dimensions can be measured accurately except in histological sections. Therefore, in order to study the growth of the very early germ, and especially the relative contribution of the soft tissue components, serial sections of histologically fixed tooth germs have been laboriously analysed, though not as yet human material. Each technique is suited to investigating a particular developmental stage of the tooth germ, the collected results depicting the overall growth picture.

From what has already been said concerning cusp development it is clear that the distances between developing cusp tips increase as the crown

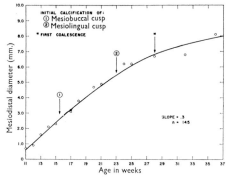

Fig. 20.—Graph of mean mesiodistal diameters of mandibular first primary molars plotted against age. (*Figs.* 20–22 *reproduced from Kraus and Jordan,* 1965.)

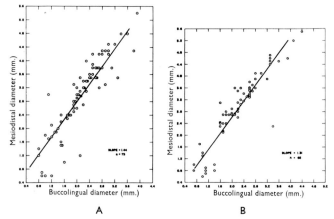

A   B

Fig. 21.—Graphs of mesiodistal diameters of, A, mandibular first primary molars and, B, mandibular second primary molars, plotted against buccolingual diameters.

becomes larger (*Fig.* 18D, E, F). It will be recalled that the cusps sometimes tilt during development and this is an additional factor determining intercuspal distance. Once the spreading front of mineralized tissue reaches the floors of the intervening valleys, the flanking dentine cusps are stabilized and their intercuspal distances remain constant (*Fig.* 18G). Any further changes in the sharpness of ridges and cusps will then be due to differences in the thickness of enamel secreted on the dentine template. Direct measurements of growth taken from series of alizarin red stained crowns of human primary lower molars show that the mesiodistal diameter of the internal enamel epithelium increases rapidly until the mineralization fronts of the mesiobuccal and distobuccal cusps unite in the floor of the intervening valley. Thereafter, the rate of increase in this diameter is greatly reduced since further growth is only due to the slow deposition of

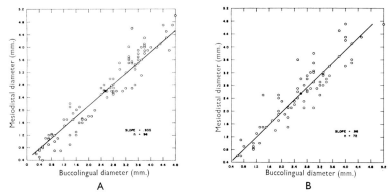

Fig. 22.—Graphs of mesiodistal diameters of, A, maxillary first primary molars and, B, maxillary second primary molars, plotted against buccolingual diameters.

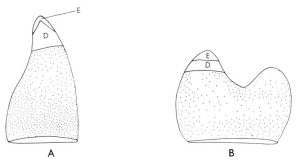

Fig. 23.—Distribution of dividing cells in the inner dental epithelium of human tooth germs. A, |B. Note the greater density of dividing cells in the cingulum zone. B, D|. Note area of dividing cells between the cusps. Not to scale. D, dentine; E, enamel.

enamel on the sides of the tooth (*Fig.* 20). It has further been shown that in these same teeth the rate of growth in the mesiodistal diameter exceeds that in the buccolingual diameter (*Fig.* 21). Hence the definitive crown is longer than it is broad. The corresponding upper primary molars grow more rapidly along the buccolingual than the mesiodistal diameter and the definitive crown is broader than long (*Fig.* 22). Similar results have been obtained from measurements of developing mouse molars. These teeth all grow very rapidly by increase in size and number of cells up to the time of completion of the crown pattern which roughly coincides with the appearance of the mineralized tissues. Thereafter, a slower rate of growth continues by accretion of enamel.

It is known that the tissue components of the developing mouse molar do not all grow at the same rate. The rate of growth of the surface area of the inner enamel epithelium is most rapid up to the time of completion of the definitive shape of the presumptive enamel-dentine junction. During this time, mitosis figures are abundant in the inner dental epithelium particularly in the presumptive cingulum zone, and growth consists essentially of cell multiplication. This is the time when the inner enamel epithelium is functioning as a surface of metabolic exchange between the enamel organ and the papilla and coincides with a maximum vascular supply to the papilla. Although little corresponding evidence is yet available for the human developing tooth, occasional references are encountered in the literature showing a similar pattern of distribution of mitosis figures, so that it is reasonable to suppose the growth processes in the different teeth to be closely comparable (*Fig.* 23). In the mouse molars the enamel organ has a slightly greater volume than the dental papilla up to the time of crown pattern completion, though both components grow at the same rate. Later, however, as the stellate reticulum becomes reduced, the enamel organ shrinks, becoming smaller than the dental papilla. Descriptive accounts, as opposed to actual measurements, suggest that the enamel organ grows rapidly in a basal direction to enshroud the papilla, but in the mouse at least it is known that this apparent enshrouding is in reality due to an overall change in shape of the inner enamel epithelium from hemispherical to conical.

This suggests that descriptive accounts of developing human teeth need to be checked by actual measurements of the component tissues of the dental organ.

In general terms, then, the present state of our knowledge enables us to say that growth of the tooth germ comprises two phases. During the first (soft tissue) phase the dental organ rapidly changes in both size and shape. Cells are rapidly dividing and morphogenetic processes are taking place. In the succeeding (hard tissue) phase the shape has already been established and there is only growth in size due to the deposition of enamel and dentine. The rate of cell division is waning and hard tissues are being deposited.

REFERENCES

BUTLER, P. M. (1968), 'Growth of the Human Second Lower Deciduous Molar', *Archs oral Biol.*, **13**, 671.

CHRISTENSEN, G. J. (1967), 'Occlusal Morphology of Human Molar Tooth Buds', *Ibid.*, **12**, 141.

GAUNT, W. A. (1963), 'An Analysis of the Growth of the Cheek Teeth of the Mouse', *Acta. Anat.*, **54**, 220.

KRAUS, B. S., and JORDAN, R. E. (1965), *see* Chapter VI.

STACK, M. V. (1964), 'A Gravimetric Study of Crown Growth Rate of the Human Deciduous Dentition', *Biol. Neonat.*, **6**, 197.

TURNER, E. P. (1963), 'Crown Development in Human Deciduous Molar Teeth', *Archs oral Biol.*, **8**, 523.

CHAPTER VIII

THE BLOOD-SUPPLY TO THE TEETH

IN studying the vascular supply to the dental tissues, it is necessary to determine the origin of the vessels, their arrangement, distribution, and density both within and around the tooth. Where tissue development is rapid there is a rich blood-supply, and the more complex the organization of the particular structure, whether anatomically or physiologically, the more abundant are the anastomoses of blood capillaries to be found. Density of the capillary network is most important in controlling the growth of the tissue, for on it depends the hypertrophy or atrophy of the tissue supplied. Abnormal blood-supply leads to hypertrophy or atrophy of the whole or parts of the tooth, irregularities of surface configuration, defects in quality of the organic or inorganic components, and other structural or physiological deviations from the typical form.

Although it is possible by laborious analysis of serial sections to reconstruct a panoramic view of vascular distribution to the teeth, the majority of investigations so far reported are based upon procedures involving the replacement of the blood in the vessels by an injected mass whose properties determine the techniques of examination subsequently employed. Coloured dyes, india ink, tinted latex, or coloured precipitates formed within the vessels by interaction between injected chemicals, all reveal the vascular architecture with great clarity, especially when combined with bulk clearing the whole specimens, rendering them transparent. In recent years, acid corrosion techniques have been developed. The surrounding tissues are removed by a corrosive fluid, leaving a three-dimensional model of the vascular system. Radio-opaque injection media enable the vascular pattern to be studied radiographically. Two new techniques have recently proved useful in studies of vascular distribution. One technique involves the use of plastic microspheres of known dimension which are injected directly into an artery and allowed to circulate. The microspheres lodge in that portion of the vascular bed where the vessels are of the same diameter as the microspheres. When histological sections are examined the plastic microspheres are clearly seen marking the vessels in which they have lodged. In this way the distribution of any selected part of the arterial system can be studied. The second technique is the histochemical demonstration of adenosine tri-phosphatase (ATP-ase) in blood-vessel walls.

Two basic difficulties are common to all injection techniques. First, the substance must be injected into fresh material under sufficient pressure to fill completely the vascular system but not so great as to rupture the vessels. This gives a picture of the entire vascular bed. However, the entire vascular bed is not fully patent at any one time during life; the pressure applied at the time of injection must certainly have opened a proportion of the smaller channels which would normally be temporarily collapsed. The second problem arises from the technical difficulty of representing a three-dimensional system on a two-dimensional picture. Though absence of the third dimension in the illustrations can be compensated for by written description, the entire complexity of the injected system can only be seen in the original model.

The few published accounts concerning blood-supply to primate and human dentitions are in broad agreement with the much more detailed investigations relating to the corresponding system in small mammals. Hence, the picture of vascular supply to the teeth presented in the following paragraphs will be a composite one.

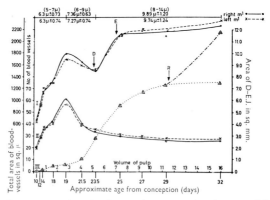

Fig. 24.—Graphs showing, I, the total cross-sectional area of blood-vessels entering the base of the dental papilla in the upper first mouse molar; II, the numbers of such vessels; and, III, the area of the enamel-dentine junction, all plotted against age. D, Time of start of dentinogenesis; E, time of start of amelogenesis; R, onset of root formation. The mean diameters of the vessels and their standard errors are also shown. (*Figs.* 24, 25 *reproduced from Gaunt*, 1960.)

The mammalian upper teeth and their supporting tissues all derive their blood-supply from branches of the superior dental arteries, supplemented to varying degrees by branches of the palatal vessels. The corresponding lower teeth and their supporting structures are supplied by branches of the inferior dental arteries which lie within the inferior dental canals; additional supply is derived from branches of the lingual vessels. As stated in Chapter IV these vessels are present in the jaws of very early cat embryos, even before the appearance of tooth germs. From these as yet thin-walled vessels capillaries arise which are concentrated along the jaws in localized regions which indicate the sites of future tooth germs. In the regions between the future tooth germs, and also in the rodent diastema, there is a sharp reduction in the capillary concentration. Such vascular arrangements have not been reported in primate or human foetal jaws, though it is very probable that here too a closely comparable situation could be demonstrated.

Reconstructions of mammalian and primate tooth germs from serial sections show that groups of blood-vessels, originating from the superior and inferior dental arteries, first pass into the dental papilla at the cap stage of development. Detailed analysis of these vessels in the mouse molars (*Fig.* 24) shows that they increase in number during the period of histo-differentiation of the tooth germ, reaching a maximum concentration immediately before the phase of most active folding of the inner dental epithelium. Gradually, with the onset of dentinogenesis, the number of vessels decreases and then becomes stabilized for that particular tooth. It will also be seen from *Fig.* 24 that the total blood-flow, computed from the mean diameters of the vessels, increases in parallel manner during this vital morphogenetic period.

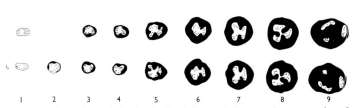

Fig. 25.—Apical views of the developing left and right second upper molar of the mouse showing the blood-vessels entering the dental papilla. Each dot represents a blood-vessel.

At no time during development do blood-vessels penetrate into the enamel organ, so that up to the start of dentinogenesis, the inner enamel epithelium probably obtains the majority of its nutrient via the papillary vessels rather than via the outer enamel epithelium.

It would thus appear that when dentine is produced it forms a barrier which prevents further metabolic exchange between the enamel organ and the dental papilla. This suggestion has received support from histo-chemical evidence and from the cytological rearrangement of the organelles within the cells of the inner enamel epithelium (*see* Chapter XV). Lying adjacent to the outer enamel epithelium is a plexus of blood-vessels which originate partly from the basal vessels before they pass into the dental papilla, and partly from the periosteal plexus associated with the developing tooth socket.

The blood-vessels passing into the dental papilla branch successively, their finest terminations pushing between the odontoblasts as capillary loops from a sub-odontoblastic plexus.

Before the roots are formed, the vessels entering the papilla congregate in groups whose number and position coincide with the number and location of the roots specific to that tooth (*Fig.* 25). It has been suggested that each of these vascular bundles supplies a separate growth centre within the papilla, though so far without conclusive evidence. As the tooth ages so the pulp chamber diminishes in volume (Chapter XXIII), the apical foramina become progressively narrowed by invading cement and the blood-supply becomes reduced. Thus it is that the tooth in old age receives but a very small proportion of its original blood-supply and the viability of the pulp diminishes.

The blood-supply to the tissues surrounding the tooth which include the periodontal ligament, the gingiva, the alveolar bone, and the epithelial attachment must now be considered.

Examination of material, utilizing the techniques already described, reveals an astonishing vascular density in the tissues adjacent to the tooth. The main supply to the ligament is via the dental artery (*Fig.* 26). This artery initially has an intrabony course and gives off alveolar branches. One enters the periodontium apically, gives off two longitudinal periodontal arteries and then continues to supply the pulp. Interalveolar arteries ascend to the crest of the alveolus giving off many perforating branches which enter the periodontal ligament at right angles to the socket wall. At the crest of the alveolus these vessels continue on to supply the

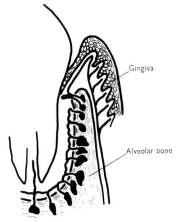

Gingiva

Alveolar bone

Fig. 26.—Diagram illustrating the arterial supply of the periodontium.

attachment epithelium and the col area. The perforating arteries are numerous and have been shown to increase in number from tooth to tooth towards the posterior teeth and, in single rooted teeth, to be greatest in number in the gingival third of the ligament and least in the middle third. The perforating arteries run parallel to the fibre bundles of the ligament and form an arcading network closer to the bone surface than to the cement surface. The classic description of longitudinal arteries running in the periodontal ligament has been questioned. When plastic microspheres are injected into the arterial system they are only found lodged in the perforating arteries. This means that either the longitudinal vessels described after injection techniques represent the venous return or are of such a diameter that the plastic microspheres do not lodge within their lumen. In view of the profuse arterial supply via the socket wall it is more than likely that the longitudinal vessels are associated with the venous drainage of the ligament.

The blood-supply to the gingiva and attachment apparatus shows distinct regional differences. The marginal and attached gingiva receive blood from vessels running in the periosteum of the alveolar process. Branches from these vessels run perpendicular to the surface and form loops within the connective tissue papillae of the gingiva. The vessels supplying the crevicular and attachment epithelium, however, show a different disposition. These are derived mainly from intrabony arteries which leave the alveolar process in the crestal area and pursue a course close to and parallel with the epithelium forming a rich network of vessels. In the region of the col, vessels leave the crest of the alveolar bone, and run perpendicularly to the surface of the col. Close to the surface they bend sharply and run parallel to the basement membrane supporting the col epithelium. The difference in the spatial arrangement of vessels in the attached gingiva and the crevicular epithelium most likely reflects the differences in the architecture of the junction between epithelium and its supporting connective tissue. In the presence of inflammation the flat junction supporting the crevicular and attachment epithelium changes and pegs of proliferative epithelium are found. At the same time the vascular supply to this region now develops looped vessels.

Thus essentially the blood-supply to the peridontium can be divided into three zones: that to the periodontal ligament, that to the gingiva facing the oral cavity, and that to the gingiva facing the tooth. However, anastomoses have been demonstrated between all three areas and this allows for a considerable collateral circulation in the supporting tissues of the tooth.

REFERENCES

BIRN, H. (1966), 'The Vascular Supply of the Periodontal Membrane', *J. periodont. Res.*, **1**, 51.

EGELBERG, J. (1966), 'The Blood Vessels of the Dentino-gingival Junction', *Ibid.*, **1**, 163.

FOLKE, L. E. A., and STALLARD, R. E. (1967), 'Periodontal Microcirculation as revealed by Plastic Microspheres', *Ibid.*, **2**, 53.

GAUNT, W. A. (1969), 'The Vascular Supply in relation to the Formation of Roots on the Cheek Teeth of the Mouse', *Acta anat.*, **43**, 116.

KINDLOVA, M. (1965), 'The Blood Supply of the Marginal Periodontium in *Macacus rhesus*', *Archs oral Biol.*, **10**, 869.

Chapter IX

COLLAGEN

Collagen is an essential constituent of connective tissue so that, apart from enamel, it is involved in all the dental tissues and plays an important part in the development, structure, and function of the tooth and its attachment apparatus. It is suggested that collagen is essential for the initiation of mineralization, that it provides the force for tooth eruption and plays an important role in the mechanism of tooth support. Therefore, some knowledge of collagen formation, structure, and breakdown is essential for a full understanding of dental histology.

The chemical composition of collagen is unique and, whilst not delving into the detailed chemistry in this book, there are certain features which are of importance and interest. The amino-acids found in collagen fall into two groups, those present in large amounts and those in small amounts. Two-thirds of the total amino-acids are represented by glycine, alanine, proline, and hydroxyproline, whilst the remaining one-third consists of fourteen other amino-acids. Two amino-acids found in collagen, hydroxyproline and hydroxylysine, are not found in other animal tissue proteins. The amino-acids of collagen are assembled together in the form of polypeptide chains consisting approximately of some 1000 amino-acid units bound together by peptide linkages. The collagen macromolecule, the building block of collagen, consists of three such polypeptide chains. Each single chain is coiled around its own axis in a simple left hand helix and the three chains, when together, are coiled like a three-stranded rope in a right hand helix. The macromolecule is synthesized by the fibroblast. This cell is characterized ultrastructurally by the presence of much rough endoplasmic reticulum and a well developed Golgi complex. The ribosomes associated with the rough endoplasmic reticulum have a characteristic spiral configuration and it is reasonably certain that the polypeptide chains are assembled at this site. How they are assembled is not known nor is the route by which they are passed out of the cell. Autoradiographic studies suggest two pathways. One from the rough endoplasmic reticulum via the Golgi complex to the exterior of the cell and the other directly to the exterior of the cell. An interesting observation in this regard is that neither hydroxyproline nor hydroxlysine is incorporated directly into the collagen macromolecule during synthesis. Proline and lysine are first incorporated and then subsequently hydroxylated. It has been shown that collagen macromolecules cannot be secreted by the cell until this hydroxylation has taken place and this may occur at the cell surface.

The collagen macromolecule, once secreted by the fibroblast, undergoes aggregation with other collagen macromolecules to form collagen fibres. The macromolecule, usually referred to as 'tropocollagen', is thus best regarded as the building block of collagen, formed within the cell but assembled into the collagen fibril extracellularly.

The mechanism whereby the collagen macromolecules are aggregated together is not certain but it probably first involves electrostatic forces between charged groups of neighbouring macromolecules. The evidence for this is as follows. Normal collagen fibrils when viewed with the electron microscope show a characteristic banding repeating at every 640 Å. If a solution of collagen macromolecules is reconstituted in 1 per cent sodium chloride a fibril repeating at 640 Å is formed. If the concentration of the electrolyte is varied collagen fibrils with a repeating band every 2800 Å are produced. This effect of the electrolyte environment on the aggregation of collagen macromolecules is consistent with the presence of electrostatic forces between macromolecules. Thus in young collagen first formed after aggregation of the macromolecules there exists a triple helix of polypeptide chains joined together by hydrogen bonds which in turn are aggregated with similar units by means of electrostatic bonds. This is an extremely unstable state and probably only exists at the initial formation of the extracellular collagen fibrils for it is known that collagen becomes progressively more stable and insoluble as collagen matures. Collagen maturation involves the formation of additional strong cross-linkages in the form of covalent bonds. These cross-linkages occur between the individual polypeptide chains and also between the collagen macromolecules.

The way in which the collagen macromolecules aggregate to give the structural basis of collagen with its characteristic 640 Å banding as seen with the electron microscope is not certain. It has been suggested that each macromolecule has five bonding zones alternating with four non-bonding zones. Such an arrangement would permit random lateral aggregation of the macromolecules producing electron dense bands at regular intervals corresponding with the bonding zones.

This account so far enables an understanding of some important experimental work done on tooth eruption which implicates collagen as providing the force which moves the tooth. This work, discussed fully in Chapter XX, involves either the use of lathyritic agents or scorbutic animals. Both result in a failure of tooth eruption and both exert their effect through collagen. In the absence of vitamin C there is a deficiency of collagen fibres. It has now been shown conclusively that vitamin C is essential for the oxidation of proline to hydroxyproline. This step occurs within the cell and in its absence the macromolecules can no longer be secreted into the extracellular environment. On the other hand, lathyritic agents interfere with collagen synthesis in an entirely different way. Lathyritic agents are nitriles of organic acids and they prevent the formation of both intra- and intermolecular cross-linkages during collagen maturation. Thus their effect is entirely extracellular.

Collagen turnover and breakdown is also significant in another context. Whilst collagen is usually thought of as being very stable, its turnover has been demonstrated by means of autoradiography in the periodontal ligament, especially in the continuously erupting rodent incisor. Collagen breakdown occurs in the connective tissue in advance of the erupting tooth and involves the enzyme collagenase. This enzyme has proved extremely difficult to demonstrate in mammalian tissue. Not only does this enzyme seem to be unstable but its action is specific and involves only an initial attack on collagen. Once this has taken place a whole series of proteolytic enzymes is capable of further breaking down collagen. Whilst bone removal is mediated by the multinucleated osteoclast, the cells involved in collagen removal and remodelling have not been indentified unequivocally. However, the most recent work in this field has implicated the fibrocyte. In the removal of a mass of collagen produced in response to an injection of foreign material, the fibroblast has been shown to undergo certain ultrastructural changes and to produce enzymes. Significantly, similar changes have been shown to occur in the fibrocytes in the connective tissue over erupting teeth. These changes involve hypertrophy of the Golgi complex and rough endoplasmic reticulum which might be indicative of increased proteolytic enzyme secretion on the part of the fibrocyte.

REFERENCES

EASTOE, J. E. (1968), 'Collagen and Tissue Architecture', *Dent. Pract. dent. Rec.*, **18**, 267.

FITTON, J. S. (1968), 'The Morphogenesis of Collagen', in *Treatise on Collagen* (ed. GOULD, B. S.), Vol. 2, part B, pp. 1–66. New York: Academic.

MELCHER, A. H., and EASTOE, J. E. (1969), 'The Connective Tissues of the Periodontium', in *The Biology of the Periodontium* (ed. MELCHER, A. H., and BOWEN, W. H.), pp. 176–343. New York: Academic.

ROSS, R. (1968), 'The Connective Tissue Fibre-forming Cell', in *Treatise on Collagen* (ed. GOULD, B. S.), vol. 2, part A, pp. 2–82. New York: Academic.

TEN CATE, A. R. (1971), 'Physiological Resorption of Connective Tissue associated with Tooth Eruption. An Electron Microscopic Study', *J. periodont. Res.*, in the press.

CHAPTER X

HARD TISSUE GENESIS

MOST accounts of hard tissue genesis deal specifically with a particular hard tissue and such accounts will also be found later in this book. The purpose of this chapter is to outline the factors common to the formation of all hard tissues and to emphasize the similar principles involved in each, though the details of structure and composition may differ considerably.

When the forming hard tissues are studied it is readily apparent that there are many common features and these are represented in diagrammatic form in *Fig.* 27. Reference to this figure reveals that, in simple terms, hard tissue genesis involves the production of an organic matrix and the

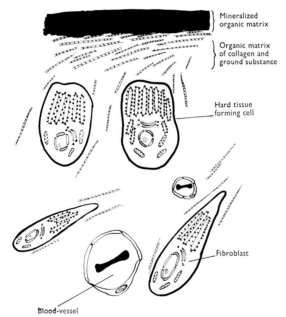

Mineralized organic matrix

Organic matrix of collagen and ground substance

Hard tissue forming cell

Fibroblast

Blood-vessel

Fig. 27.—Diagram showing the essential features of hard tissue genesis.

introduction into this matrix of mineral salts. The first step, therefore, in producing any hard tissue is to elaborate the organic matrix and for this a specialized cell is required. Such cells differentiate in areas of marked vascularity and have well defined characteristics. Histochemically a marked RNA content can be demonstrated together with a high oxidative enzyme activity and a high hydrolytic enzyme activity. Ultrastructural features include a well developed 'rough' endoplasmic reticulum, Golgi apparatus, numerous mitochondrea and secretory vesicles. These histochemical and ultrastructural features indicate that these are protein-synthesizing and secreting cells. The proteins they secrete are built up extracellularly into a fibrous form which constitutes the fibrous component of the organic matrix. The organic matrix of hard tissue consists also of a cementing or ground substance lying between the fibres, of which two essential constituents are acid mucopolysaccharides and carbohydrate-containing proteins. Ground substance is derived from the activity of the cells already described but can also be provided by other cells found in close association with the protein secreting cell. At this stage it is confusing to discuss this controversial point further and it is best to accept for the time being the presence of ground substance as an essential constituent of the organic matrix.

It is unfortunate that obscurity exists concerning the mechanism whereby mineral salts are introduced into an organic matrix. The present consensus of opinion is that mineralization occurs by 'seeding' of the organic matrix, that is, 'planting of seeds' or the initiation of nuclei of crystallization within the organic matrix; further mineralization occurs by epitaxy, which means the layered overgrowth of one crystal on another. The seed or nucleus which initiates epitaxy may also be called the 'epitactic focus'. A good analogy here is the well-known experiment in which crystals are induced to grow by introducing dust particles ('planting seeds') into a super-saturated solution of copper sulphate: each dust particle acts as a nucleus of crystallization on which there is a subsequent layered overgrowth of crystals (epitaxy). However, *in vitro* experiments show that crystals form spontaneously providing that the concentration of Ca and PO_4 ions is sufficiently high. *In vivo* nucleating substances of unknown composition are present around which crystals form at physiological concentrations of Ca and PO_4 ions, considerably less than those required in the *in vitro* systems, and once crystal growth has begun it will continue at even lower concentrations.

Recent studies of hard tissue genesis using the techniques of inert dehydration, which preserves extracellular material well, and electron microscopy, are of interest concerning the mechanism whereby mineral salts are introduced into an organic matrix. These studies suggest that at all sites of initial mineralization the cell concerned buds to provide the epitactic foci. This possible cellular involvement would explain why it is that the organic matrix of hard tissues, as distinct from other forms of connective tissue, permits mineralization. Further reference to these studies will be made as the genesis of each hard tissue is discussed for it seems that there is a significant difference in the method of mineralization dependent upon whether mineralization is taking place *de novo*, or in relationship to pre-existing mineralized tissue.

The association of the activity of the enzyme alkaline phosphatase (a hydrolytic enzyme) with the genesis of hard tissue has been established for many years. It was first thought that the activity of this enzyme was concerned with mineralization, but the weight of evidence at the present time indicates that the enzyme's activity is concerned with the elaboration of the organic matrix. This is a point which will be discussed further in relation to dentinogenesis as in this case there is a pertinent pointer to its function in the production of the organic matrix.

The marked activity of other hydrolytic enzymes (especially acid phosphatase) in hard tissue forming cells has not yet been related to any specific function. Indeed, acid phosphatase activity is usually associated with catabolic events, and it is therefore somewhat surprising to find high activity of this enzyme in a cell primarily associated with anabolism.

Having outlined in fairly simple terms the salient features of hard tissue genesis, it is a rewarding exercise to examine the formation of the individual hard tissues to see how closely they are comparable. At the same time such a comparison should emphasize the similar principles involved in the genesis of each tissue.

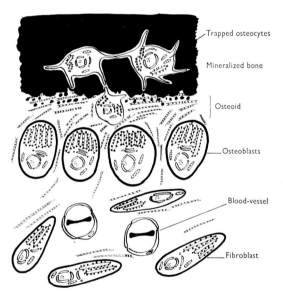

Fig. 28.—Diagrammatic representation of osteogenesis.

The formation of bone is described as taking place by two methods, intramembranous or endochondral. Both methods are fundamentally the same because, although in endochondral bone formation the bone is preceded by a cartilaginous model, this is replaced by bone deposited in the same way as in the intramembranous situation. Bone is a mineralized connective tissue and its formation (intramembranous bone formation) is heralded by an increase in local vascularity of the mesenchyme. At the same time the cells of the mesenchyme in this area differentiate into distinctive cells called 'osteoblasts'. These cells are rich in RNA, associated with a well developed 'rough' endoplasmic reticulum, have a well developed Golgi apparatus, and show high hydrolytic and oxidative enzyme activity. They synthesize the ground substance and the forerunners of the collagen macromolecule (tropocollagen) which is assembled extracellularly into collagen fibres in the ground substance. The collagen fibres and the ground substance constitute the organic matrix of unmineralized bone (osteoid), and it is into this that mineral salts are deposited. The first foci of mineral salts in the organic matrix are related to protoplasmic buds of the osteoblasts. Continued crystal growth from these foci results in the osteoblast becoming surrounded by mineralized matrix and the cell is then termed an 'osteocyte'. *Fig.* 28 illustrates this sequence of events and it will be seen that it is essentially similar to *Fig.* 27, differing only in that the bone-forming cells become trapped within the forming hard tissue. In endochondral bone formation the disintegrating cartilage model is invaded by vascular mesenchymal osteogenic tissue which elaborates bone in essentially the same manner as outlined above. There is one significant difference,

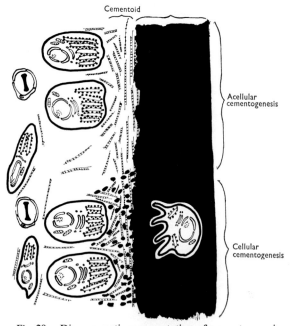

Fig. 29.—Diagrammatic representation of cementogenesis.

however; as the cartilage model is invaded by osteogenic tissue the cartilage mineralizes and this mineralized cartilage provides the scaffold for the forming bone. In this situation the newly formed osteoid does not seem to mineralize from epitactic foci provided by osteoblastic buds. Instead mineralization occurs by crystal growth from the pre-existing crystallites in the mineralized cartilage. It must be pointed out that this account of bone formation applies to the formation of embryonic bone. The coarse-fibred embryonic bone later undergoes remodelling to be replaced by adult fine-fibred bone.

The mode of formation of cement is almost identical to that of bone. Cement is also a mineralized connective tissue and is formed by cementoblasts, the cement-forming cells, which differentiate from the ectomesenchymal part of the dental follicle surrounding the developing root. These cells exhibit high hydrolytic enzyme activity, oxidative enzyme activity, and have a well developed 'rough' endoplasmic reticulum and Golgi apparatus. They elaborate the collagen fibres of the unmineralized cement matrix (cementoid). The cementoblasts may or may not be incorporated in the mineralizing matrix and this determines the two types of cement seen in

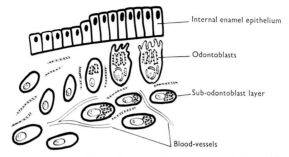

Fig. 30.—Diagram illustrating the differentiation of odontoblasts.

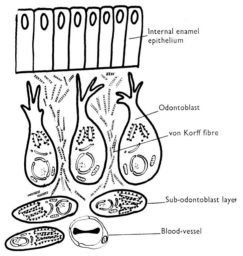

Fig. 31.—Diagram illustrating the origin and distribution of the classic von Korff fibre.

histological sections, acellular and cellular. *Fig.* 29 gives the essential details of cementogenesis. As cement is laid down over the pre-existing dentine, the initial mineralization of the cementoid takes place by crystal growth from the mineralized dentine.

Like cement, dentine is also formed from ectomesenchymal connective tissue but it differs significantly from bone and cement, especially in its structural features. Even so the principles underlying its formation are the same. Specialized cells, the odontoblasts, differentiate from the cells of the dental papilla due to induction by the cells of the internal enamel epithelium. At the same time other papillary cells congregate beneath the newly differentiated odontoblasts, forming the sub-odontoblast layer (*Fig.* 30) between which are the vessels of the sub-odontoblast capillary plexus. The newly differentiated odontoblasts develop an extensive endoplasmic reticulum, a prominent Golgi apparatus, and exhibit marked oxidative and hydrolytic enzyme activity apart from alkaline phosphatase. This enzyme is found initially in the cells of the sub-odontoblast layer and it is from this layer that large fibre bundles, the fibres of von Korff,

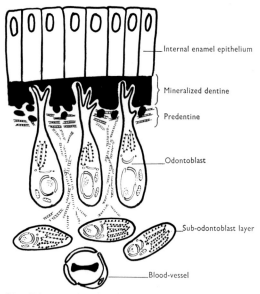

Fig. 32.—Diagram showing the formation of dentinal tubules.

originate. These fibres pass between the odontoblasts and fan out close to the basement membrane of the internal enamel epithelium and, together with the ground substance, constitute the organic matrix of the first formed dentine (*Fig.* 31). While the organic matrix is being formed, the odontoblasts retreat towards the centre of the papilla each leaving behind a slender process which becomes surrounded by matrix. The dentine matrix becomes mineralized to form tubular dentine (*Fig.* 32). The technique of inert dehydration reveals that the odontoblasts in this situation like the osteoblasts in membranous ossification, have cellular buds which provide the foci for mineralization. This sequence of events only applies to the very first dentine (mantle dentine) elaborated against the internal enamel epithelium. After this first increment of dentine forms, the fibrous component for the remainder of the matrix is manufactured by the odontoblasts (*Fig.* 33). It is significant that when this switch in the origin of the fibrous matrix occurs, there is a reduction in the number of von Korff fibres and the enzyme alkaline phosphatase now becomes demonstrable within the odontoblasts. This widely accepted account of dentinogenesis is correct in principal. However, very recent studies have queried whether von Korff fibres really exist and these studies will be discussed fully in the chapter on dentinogenesis.

Thus far, therefore, it is evident that osteogenesis, cementogenesis, and dentinogenesis have many common features. These hard tissues are all specialized forms of connective tissue; they all develop in areas of high vascularity; specialized cells are associated with the formation of the organic matrix which consists of collagen fibres and a ground substance. The cells have common ultrastructural and enzymatic features and mineralization occurs within the organic matrix.

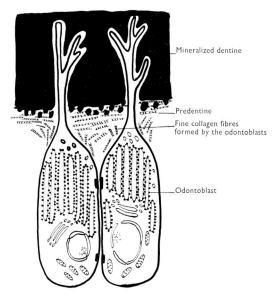

Fig. 33.—Diagram illustrating circumpulpal dentinogenesis.

When amelogenesis is considered, it would appear that enamel formation differs significantly from that of the other hard tissues. Enamel is an ectodermal product and for this reason its organic matrix cannot contain the strictly mesenchymal or ectomesenchymal product collagen. By analogy with the fibrous collagen scaffolding of other mesenchymal hard tissues, it was once assumed that enamel employed a fibrous protein, keratin, to fulfil the same function. However, this is now known not to be the case and, although no fibrous component is involved in enamel matrix formation, amelogenesis can be shown to be closely similar in principle to the formation of other hard tissues.

The histology of amelogenesis outlined in *Fig.* 34 shows that two cellular elements are involved, the enamel forming cells or ameloblasts, and the cells of the stratum intermedium. The latter are exceptionally rich in alkaline phosphatase activity and the ameloblasts are rich in RNA and have a high activity of oxidative enzymes. If the ultrastructure of the ameloblast is examined, its features are essentially similar to those of the osteoblast or odontoblast in that there is a well developed 'rough' endoplasmic reticulum, Golgi apparatus, many mitochondria and secretory vesicles. In other words, it has the characteristics of a protein synthesizing and secreting cell.

In view of the once supposed presence of keratinous material in enamel matrix, it is interesting to compare the ultrastructure of the ameloblast with that of the keratin producing cell. The keratinizing cell has very little 'rough' endoplasmic reticulum and instead has many free ribosomes.

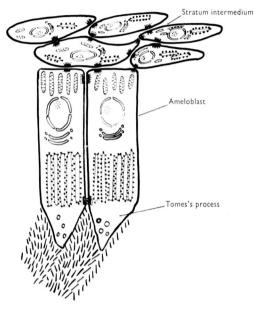

Stratum intermedium

Ameloblast

Tomes's process

Fig. 34.—Diagram illustrating the cells associated with amelogenesis.

The protein synthesized in this cell is retained and aggregated in a fibrous form, so that the cytoplasm eventually becomes laden with keratin. Such a cell is described as a protein-synthesizing and retaining cell and it is clear from a comparison between *Figs.* 9 and 34 that the ameloblast does not fall into this category. Thus far amelogenesis corresponds to the genesis of the other hard tissues. Blood-vessels are present, adjacent to the outer dental epithelium, the enzymatic picture corresponds, and the formative cell secretes a proteinaceous material which forms the organic matrix. However, when discussing amelogenesis later in this book, evidence will be presented showing that this organic matrix does not become organized into a fibrous form but remains in the form of a gel. Into this organic matrix mineral salts are deposited. The studies utilizing inert dehydration show that there is no evidence for any buds or protrusions associated with the ameloblast and that initial mineralization of enamel starts by crystal growth from the mineralized dentine which supports the first formed enamel matrix.

It is apparent, then, that the hard tissues, irrespective of their derivation, reveal similar principles in their genesis. These may be summarized as the production of an organic matrix by cells which exhibit protein synthesizing and secreting features, and introduction into this matrix of mineral salts.

It is useful to summarize here the new concept of mineralization of hard tissues. The suggestion is that where mineralization is occurring for the first time, such as in membranous bone formation, dentine formation, and in mineralizing cartilage, the foci for initial appearance of inorganic crystals are buds or extensions of the cell associated with deposition of the organic matrix. Where hard tissue genesis is taking place in association with pre-existing mineralized tissue, for example, cement in relation to mineralized dentine, bone in relation to mineralized cartilage, and enamel in relation to mineralized dentine, mineralization occurs in the newly formed matrix by crystal growth from the pre-existing mineralized tissue. Whilst this concept is too new to have been critically assessed, it has a sound morphological basis and needs only chemical substantiation.

REFERENCES

References pertinent to this chapter can be found following the Chapters on Dentinogenesis, Amelogenesis, and Cementogenesis.

CHAPTER XI

BONE

THE organization and structure of bone as a tissue can be a little difficult to understand because of the varying terminologies used. An extensive terminology exists because of the different ways of looking at bone. Thus descriptions of bone are based on the nature of the fibrous matrix, on the macroscopic appearance, and on the ratio of hard tissue to associated soft connective tissue. With common usage some of these terms have become intermixed, leading to confusion. In this chapter, therefore, some concepts

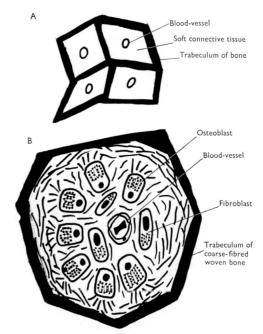

Fig. 35.—Diagram of embryonic bone formation. A, Trabeculae of bone are laid down in soft connective tissue round a central vessel or vessels. B, Detail of soft connective tissue core.

are presented which it is hoped will help in forming a clearer picture of this specialized connective tissue.

When bone tissue is first formed or when it is rapidly laid down, for example in the embryo and in the repair of wounds, the pre-existing connective tissue of the area is colonized by new bone. The pre-existing collagen in the connective tissue and the new collagen elaborated by the osteoblasts together form the fibrous matrix of this new bone. As a result the collagen fibres are of varying thickness and orientation and many are continuous with the collagen fibres of the adjacent soft connective tissue. This type of bone is termed 'coarse-fibred woven bone' or 'embryonic bone' and is laid down in trabeculae or plates which surround areas of soft connective tissue (*Fig.* 35). From this starting point bone is remodelled to form fine-fibred mature bone. In mature bone the collagen fibres of the matrix are of even thickness and are laid down in sheets or lamellae. In each lamella the collagen fibres are all orientated in one direction, although the orientation of collagen fibres varies from lamella to lamella. Lamellae

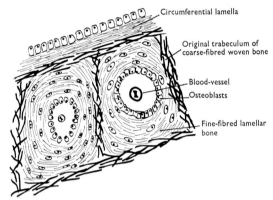

Fig. 36.—Diagram showing the formation of primary osteons within trabeculae of woven bone.

of bone are laid down in two ways. They can be laid down concentrically around blood-vessels to form osteons (Haversian systems) or in sheets on the surface of bones as circumferential lamellae. Woven bone is converted to mature bone as follows. Within the trabeculae of woven bone is soft connective tissue with associated blood-vessels. On the internal surface of the trabeculae new bone is laid down in layers or lamellae with the result that, as each layer is laid down, the volume of the soft connective tissue is diminished until only a small core of connective tissue transmitting blood-vessels remains. This osteon formed within woven bone is termed a 'primary' osteon (*Fig.* 36). The primary osteon has a periphery which is ill defined when viewed in the light microscope because the collagen fibres here are continuous with those of the woven bone. Also the cells, the osteocytes, are larger and have an irregular disposition. Thus we now have an immature form of bone which consists of a mixture of woven bone and primary osteons arranged as comparatively large trabeculae.

From this point on either mature compact bone or mature cancellous bone is developed. These two types of bone are distinguished on the ratio of hard tissue and soft connective tissue. Thus compact bone consists of comparatively solid blocks of bone in which the proportion of mineralized tissue is far greater than the proportion of soft connective tissue, whereas in cancellous bone the blocks of bone are separated by a considerable portion of soft connective tissue and macroscopically have a honeycomb appearance. Mature bone is formed by a process of remodelling where resorption first takes place indiscriminantly within the trabeculae of primary osteons and woven bone. The area resorbed is replaced by soft connective tissue. Within the concavity of the resorbed area bone is laid down in a similar manner as described for the primary osteon to form what is termed the 'secondary osteon' (*Fig.* 37). The secondary osteon is marked

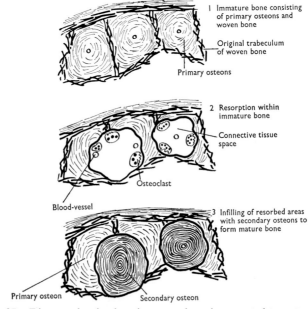

Fig. 37.—Diagram showing how immature bone is converted to mature bone.

at its periphery by a reversal line which marks the extent of resorption. Depending on the amount of remodelling and infilling of the soft connective tissue spaces either mature cancellous or mature compact bone is formed. It is important to realize that transitional forms of bone are often seen. Thus although both mature compact bone and cancellous bone are made up of secondary osteons and circumferential lamellae, both can contain primary osteons until remodelling processes eliminate and replace these by secondary osteons. Where bone is actively being remodelled, for example in the alveolar process, complete replacement by secondary osteons may never occur. During remodelling, remnants of previous osteons remain and these are termed 'interstitial bone'.

CHAPTER XII

DENTINOGENESIS

THE formation of dentine begins at the late bell stage of tooth development and is a product of the dental papilla. Immediately before the start of dentinogenesis changes are found within the cells of the internal enamel epithelium. The short columnar cells of this epithelium become tall columnar and their nuclei move to the ends of the cells away from the papilla. Tissue culture studies have shown unequivocally that these elongated cells organize the differentiation of the peripheral cells of the dental papilla into odontoblasts. However, in terms of induction, the

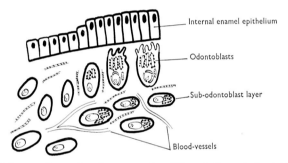

Fig. 38.—Diagram illustrating the progressive differentiation of odontoblasts from left to right.

significance of these morphological changes in the internal enamel epithelium may have been over-emphasized for a similar inductive mechanism exists between dental epithelium and papilla during root formation without the epithelial cells undergoing these changes.

The newly differentiated odontoblast is characterized histologically by its size; histochemically by its high RNA content, carbohydrate content, and marked oxidative and hydrolytic enzyme activity. This latter characteristic must be qualified in that whereas increase in acid phosphatase and esterase activity can be demonstrated, the newly differentiated odontoblast does not exhibit alkaline phosphatase activity. Ultrastructurally this cell exhibits a well developed 'rough' endoplasmic reticulum, Golgi apparatus, numerous mitochondria, many vesicular structures, and microtubules. At the same time as the odontoblasts differentiate there is an increase in the number of cells of the papilla immediately subjacent to the odontoblasts and a sub-odontoblast layer is formed. A feature of the cells of this layer is their high alkaline phosphatase activity. Between the cells is a rich capillary plexus (*Fig.* 38). Ground substance surrounds all these cellular elements.

The next step in the formation of dentine is the production of tropocollagen by the cellular elements of the sub-odontoblast layer. The tropocollagen molecules link together extracellularly so that distinct fibre bundles can be recognized at this time in silver stained sections examined with the light microscope (*Fig.* 39). These fibre bundles, the fibres of von Korff, appear to spiral between the odontoblasts and are described as fanning out against the surface of the basement lamina of the internal enamel epithelium where they form the fibrillar component of the organic matrix of the first formed dentine. Simultaneously with the formation of the von

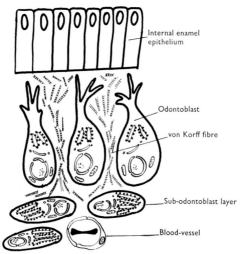

Fig. 39.—Diagram illustrating the origin and distribution of the classic von Korff fibre.

Korff fibres, the odontoblasts and the sub-odontoblast cells move away from the basement membrane. As they do so, the odontoblasts each leave behind a slender cytoplasmic odontoblast process which eventually lies within a dentine tubule when the dentine matrix becomes mineralized (*Fig.* 40).

The fibrous nature of von Korff fibres has recently been questioned. There is strong evidence that von Korff fibres are structures visible only with the light microscope. Tooth germs are stained in bulk with a silver stain and then prepared for electron microscopy. Thick sections cut for orientation purposes and examined with the light microscope show the classic appearance of von Korff fibres where initial dentinogenesis is taking place. When thin sections of the same area are examined with the electron microscope von Korff fibres are not seen. Instead the silver stain is seen as small particles filling the tissue fluid spaces between the newly differentiated odontoblasts. This 'compartment' is occupied by ground substance and a few fine non-banded fibrils. These fine fibres are so small that it is impossible to resolve them with the light microscope (*Fig.* 41). How then can this electron microscopic picture be correlated with the light microscopic picture? Studies on forming connective tissue have suggested that the branched argyrophilic reticulin seen with the light microscope may represent no more than the compartment between cells seen at the electron microscope level. A wide extracellular compartment separates the newly formed odontoblasts. This becomes impregnated with silver and when viewed with the light microscope gives a negative outline of the odontoblasts and a simulated fibrous structure (*Fig.* 42).

The origin of the ground substance of the dentine matrix has not yet been fully elucidated. Ground substance contains two characteristic

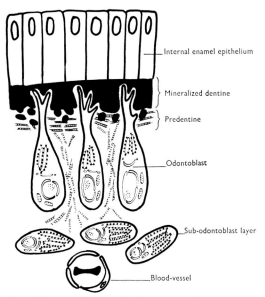

Internal enamel epithelium

Mineralized dentine

Predentine

Odontoblast

Sub-odontoblast layer

Blood-vessel

Fig. 40.—Diagram showing the formation of dentinal tubules.

components, acid mucopolysaccharides and carbohydrate-containing proteins. Mucopolysaccharides are largely carbohydrate, whereas carbohydrate-containing proteins contain a higher proportion of protein. It is known from histochemical and autoradiographic studies that during dentinogenesis acid mucopolysaccharides progressively disappear from the papilla adjacent to the odontoblasts. Also the acid mucopolysaccharide content of the papilla progressively diminishes with continued dentine formation. This suggests that the acid mucopolysaccharide component of the dentine matrix could be incorporated from the papilla. It has been shown that during the formation of dentine matrix, there is an influx of a carbohydrate component of the ground substance which obscures collagen fibres, even with the high resolution of the electron microscope. It is likely that this carbohydrate-containing protein is produced by the odontoblasts. The von Korff 'fibres' and the ground substance together form the organic matrix of the dentine which in its non-mineralized state is termed 'predentine'. It will be appreciated that there is always a layer of predentine present during dentinogenesis into which mineral salts are deposited. The principles of mineralization have already been discussed in Chapter X and these also apply to dentinogenesis. After sufficient predentine has been formed, nuclei of crystallization appear in the matrix. As with the initial mineralization of woven bone, the foci of mineralization have been linked with pseudopodial extensions or 'buds' of the odontoblast in the very first instance, with subsequent mineralization spreading from these foci.

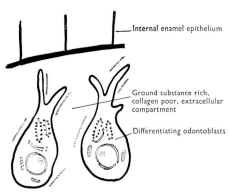

Fig. 41.—Diagram illustrating the electron microscope appearance of newly differentiated odontoblasts and the associated extracellular compartment.

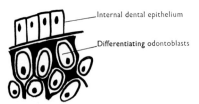

Fig. 42.—Diagram showing how silver staining of extracellular material gives the appearance of 'fibres' when examined with the light microscope.

It must be made clear that all the foregoing applies to the first dentine formed in the tooth germ, and that later dentinogenesis differs in some aspects of its formation. It has long been known that the dentine immediately below the enamel, the first formed dentine, differs from the bulk of the dentine in having an organic matrix with coarse collagen fibres. Thus mantle dentine (the first formed) and circumpulpal dentine (the bulk of the dentine) are recognized. Evidence for this duality of dentine has increased greatly over the last few years. Histologically a diminution in the number of von Korff 'fibres' has been noted when later sections of dentinogenesis are studied. Electron microscopy and autoradiography have now established with certainty that the odontoblast elaborates the fine fibred collagen of the circumpulpal dentine in place of the coarse fibres incorporated in mantle dentine (*Fig.* 43).

This dimunition in von Korff 'fibres' can now be explained on the basis of the studies described previously in this chapter. When the same method is used to study later dentinogenesis, the electron microscope shows that the odontoblasts are tightly packed together and that there is no extracellular compartment between them. Hence there is no deposition of silver and von Korff 'fibres' cannot be seen under the light microscope.

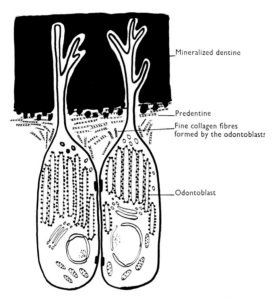

Fig. 43.—Diagram illustrating circumpulpal dentinogenesis.

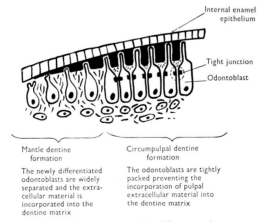

Fig. 44.—Diagram illustrating the essential differences between mantle dentine formation and circumpulpal dentine formation.

The distribution of the activity of the enzyme alkaline phosphatase has been correlated with the supposed dual origin of dentine collagen. During mantle dentine formation the activity of this enzyme is localized to the sub-odontoblast layer only. In later dentinogenesis activity of this enzyme develops in the odontoblasts. However, the function of this enzyme in the production of mineralized connective tissue has not yet been explained. Whilst there is evidence that its activity is linked with the production of organic matrix the point at issue is whether the enzyme is concerned with the synthesis of collagen or the synthesis of ground substance. If alkaline phosphatase activity is associated with ground

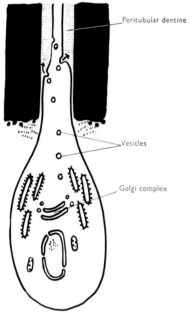

Peritubular dentine

Vesicles

Golgi complex

Fig. 45.—Diagram showing the formation of peri-tubular dentine.

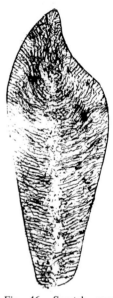

Fig. 46.—Scratch marks made on smoked card by beads simulating the primary curvatures of dentine tubules.

substance synthesis its shift in localization can be equated with differences in the formation of mantle and circumpulpal dentine. Thus, in mantle dentine formation, a good deal of ground substance rich, collagen-poor extracellular material is incorporated into the dentine matrix. When the odontoblasts become tightly packed this extracellular material is no longer available and the dentine matrix must result from odontoblastic activity only (*Fig.* 44).

Examination of the fine structure of dentine reveals the presence of a sheath of more highly mineralized peri-tubular dentine around the odontoblast process (*Fig.* 45). The first appearance of the peri-tubular dentine is in the fully mineralized dentine matrix near the predentine-dentine border and coincides with the narrowing in width of the odontoblast process; the peri-tubular dentine thus occupies some of the space formerly occupied by the odontoblast process. Little is known about the genesis of the peri-tubular dentine. However, there are certain features of the odontoblast, its process, and the peri-tubular dentine which permit some speculation. It is known that the newly formed peri-tubular dentine has a high acid mucopolysaccharide content. From studies of other cells synthesizing mucopolysaccharides, it is now clear that the Golgi apparatus is actively associated with the combination of the protein synthesized on the 'rough' endoplasmic reticulum with the carbohydrate moiety. From the Golgi apparatus this material is then passed to the cell surface in vesicular structures, which fuse with the cell membrane and thus disgorge this material into the extracellular environment. The odontoblast has a well developed Golgi apparatus and vesicular structures have been described in the odontoblast process. At the structural level, therefore, there

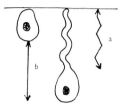

Fig. 47.—Distance a, the true length of the forming odontoblast process, is greater than b, the distance moved by the odontoblast in the same time.

is evidence which suggests that the peri-tubular acid mucopolysaccharides are synthesized within the odontoblast cell-body and transported, via the odontoblast process, to the site of peri-tubular dentine formation. Very recent studies using electron microscopic autoradiography have traced the route of tritiated proline through the functional odontoblast. After its initial location in the 'rough' endoplasmic reticulum the proline passes to the Golgi apparatus and then to the odontoblast process packaged in dense granules. The proline finally becomes localized extracellularly by passing through the cell membrane of the odontoblast process and into the peri-tubular space. It is reasonable to assume, therefore, that a similar pathway may exist for the secretion of carbohydrate material. Also within the odontoblast process during dentine formation are acid phosphatase containing lysosome-like bodies and microtubules. The functional implications of these two structures is not clear at this time.

Another interesting aspect of dentinogenesis is the course taken by the odontoblasts as they retreat towards the centre of the pulp. As they leave behind them a process which is incorporated in the mineralized matrix, examination of the tubules of mature dentine provides a permanent record of the path taken by the individual odontoblasts. It is known that the odontoblast processes have a primary 'S' shaped curvature and also secondary curvatures.

There is a hypothesis to explain the genesis of these curvatures. It has been suggested that the primary curvatures result from the oscillations of the odontoblasts which arise from their crowding as the volume of the pulp decreases. This has been tested by a simple model experiment. The outline of the dentine surface of a tooth in longitudinal section is traced on smoked paper. If beads, representing the odontoblasts, are alined along the periphery of the drawing and progressively pushed in a centripetal direction, starting with those beneath the cusp tip, the sinuous tracks so produced on the smoked paper mimic the primary curvatures of the dentinal tubules (*Fig.* 46). At the same time, it will be seen that the beads become progressively more crowded as they move centripetally. The origin of the secondary curvatures is more difficult to explain, but a tentative solution has been offered. This is based upon the accepted observation that enamel spindles are most frequently encountered beneath the tips of cusps, where crowding of the retreating odontoblasts is most intense. Under such conditions, it is suggested that in unit time the formed length of the odontoblast process is greater than the distance moved by the odontoblast towards the papilla (*Fig.* 47). Hence, the process might become buckled and the secondary curvatures established.

REFERENCES

FRANK, R. M. (1970), '*Étude autoradiographique de la dentinogenèse en microscopie electronique de l'aide de la proline tritiée chez le chat*', *Archs oral Biol.*, **15**, 583.

GARANT, P. R., ZABO, G., and NALBANDIAN, J. (1968), 'The Fine Structure of the Mouse Odontoblast', *Ibid.*, **13**, 857.

HARROP, T. J., and MACKAY, B. (1968), 'Electron Microscopic Observations on Healing in the Dental Pulp in the Rat', *Ibid.*, **13**, 365.

HEROLD, R. C., and KAYE, H. (1966), 'Mitochondria in Odontoblastic Processes', *Nature, Lond.*, **210**, 108.

LESTER, K. S., and BOYDE, A. (1968), 'The Question of von Korff Fibres in Mammalian Dentine', *Calc. Tiss. Res.*, **1**, 273.

MELCHER, A. H., and EASTOE, J. E. (1969), 'The Connective Tissues of the Periodontium', in *The Biology of the Periodontium*, (ed. MELCHER, A. H., and BOWEN, W. H.), pp. 176–343. New York: Academic.

NOBLE, H. W., CARMICHEAL, A. F., and RANKINE, H. (1962), 'Electron Microscopy of Human Developing Dentine', *Archs oral Biol.*, **7**, 395.

OSBORN, J. W. (1967), 'A Mechanistic View of Dentinogenesis and its Relation to the Curvatures of the Processes of the Odontoblasts', *Ibid.*, **12**, 275.

REITH, E. J. (1968a), 'Collagen Formation in Developing Molar Teeth of Rats', *J. Ult. Res.*, **21**, 383.

— — (1968b), 'Ultrastructural Aspects of Dentinogenesis', in *Dentine and Pulp* (ed. SYMONS, N. B. B.), pp. 19–42. Edinburgh: Livingstone.

SYMONS, N. B. B. (1956), 'The Development of the Fibres of the Dentine Matrix', *Br. dent. J.*, **101**, 252.

— — (1962), 'A Histochemical Study of the Odontoblast Process', *Archs oral Biol*, **7**, 455.

TEN CATE, A. R. (1962), 'The Distribution of Alkaline Phosphatase in the Human Tooth Germ', *Ibid.*, **7**, 195.

— — (1966), 'Alkaline Phosphatase Activity and the Formation of Human Circumpulpal Dentine, *Ibid.*, **11**, 267.

— — (1967), 'A Histochemical Study of the Human Odontoblast,' *Ibid.*, **12**, 963.

— — (1968), 'Current Concepts and Problems of Dentinogenesis', in *Dentine and Pulp* (ed. SYMONS, N. B. B.), pp. 9–18. Edinburgh: Livingstone.

— — MELCHER, A. H., PUDY, G., and WAGNER, D. (1971), 'The Non-fibrous Nature of the von Korff Fibres in Developing Dentine. A Light and Electron Microscopic Study', *Anat. Rec.*, in the press.

CHAPTER XIII

THE STRUCTURE OF DENTINE

WELL documentated accounts of dentine structure are available in the standard dental texts and no useful purpose would be served by repeating their contents. There are, however, certain structural features which have recently been investigated and it is the purpose of this chapter to present these to the reader. Some of these features are represented diagrammatically in *Fig.* 48.

The layer of dentine adjacent to the enamel (mantle dentine) differs from the bulk of the dentine (circumpulpal dentine) in the configuration of the collagen fibres of the matrix. Classically the thick fibres of von Korff are thought to form the fibre content of the mantle dentine matrix and, apart from where they fan out at the enamel dentine junction, to be parallel to the dentinal tubules. The matrix fibres of circumpulpal dentine are much finer and weave across each other at right angles to the tubules. As von Korff fibres can be seen between odontoblasts forming circumpulpal dentine it might seem that these fibres should be visible in mineralized circumpulpal dentine. However, such fibres are only rarely seen and it has been suggested that these thick fibres become split and re-orientated at right angles to the tubules during circumpulpal dentinogenesis. However, in view of the recent findings concerning von Korff fibres discussed in the previous chapter their contribution to the matrix of mantle dentine must be re-assessed. It is clear from *Fig.* 44 that as mantle dentine forms a good deal of ground substance, rich, collagen-poor extracellular material is incorporated whereas little ground substance is incorporated from the pulp into the circumpulpal dentine matrix. There is, therefore, a real difference between the matrices of mantle and circumpulpal dentine but it cannot be attributed to the presence or absence of von Korff fibres. The capricious demonstration of von Korff fibres during circumpulpal dentinogenesis at the light microscope level can be explained on the basis of the separation of some odontoblasts, the majority of which, when seen with the electron microscope, are closely packed and united by means of tight junctions. Silver deposition between the separated odontoblasts will be seen as von Korff fibres with the light microscope. In the subsurface zone of the root dentine the finer fibres are curved and said to be arranged in arcades. It is possible that as the calcospherites form they mould the fibres into these arcades which are then stabilized by the ensuing mineralization.

The highly mineralized peri-tubular dentine appears to be present in all mammalian dentines. It is generally thickest on the side of the tubule towards the occlusal surface of the tooth. Most studies have suggested that the matrix of peri-tubular dentine consists of very sparse fine collagen fibres, although it has also been suggested that this region is devoid of any fibrous material, thus giving it affinities with enamel. Recent electron microscope studies show that there is a space between the odontoblast process and the tubule wall; this space is termed the 'periodontoblastic space'. These same studies showed that the space was occupied by an amorphous ground substance containing occasional fine non-mineralized collagen fibres, which may or may not become incorporated in the hyper-mineralized peri-tubular dentine. Electron micrographs have recently shown the presence of one or more thick non-mineralized collagen fibres running beside the odontoblast process within the dentine tubule. Though

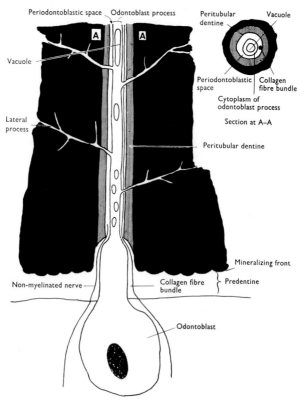

Fig. 48.—Diagram showing some of the features thought to exist in relation to the odontoblast process. Not to scale.

their presence is as yet unexplained, it might be that they are produced by aggregation of the fine collagen fibres just mentioned.

An explanation of the origin of the primary and secondary curvatures of the dentine tubules has been proposed in the previous chapter. Phase contrast and electron microscopic examinations of human dentine reveal that large numbers of lateral processes arise from, and are directly con-tinuous with, the odontoblast processes. These branches run towards those from adjacent systems and permeate the dentine matrix though there is no evidence of protoplasmic continuity between them. The lateral processes are protoplasmic and must be formed at the level of the pulp-predentine junction, being subsequently caught up in the advancing front of the mineralizing dentine. It is conceivable that they form the anatomical pathways for the transport of materials between the odontoblast processes and the more distant parts of the matrix. They may even direct the formation of their own investing matrix deep within the dentine, although there is no evidence to support this.

From time to time cytoplasmic vacuoles within the odontoblasts have been described. Recent electron microscopic studies show that these vacuoles are also present within the odontoblast process, being relatively small and quite numerous at the pulpal end but becoming large, elongated, and less numerous in the direction of the enamel-dentine junction. In the latter region, they appear to occupy the majority of the odontoblastic process, squeezing the cytoplasm of the process into a narrow peripheral zone. The contents of the vacuoles appear finely stippled under the electron microscope and this material is thought to be discharged into the peri-odontoblastic space by a process of reverse pinocytosis. However, the chemical nature of the vacuole contents has not yet been investigated. At these high magnifications, the cytoplasm of the most terminal end of the odontoblast processes has a hyaline appearance. Recent histochemical studies show the presence of hydrolytic enzymes and lipid, represented in particulate form, within the odontoblast process and the lateral processes. Their localization may possibly correspond with the vacuolar structures seen in electron micrographs suggesting that the odontoblast process is not merely an inactive cell extension. A few mitochondria have now been demonstrated in the odontoblast process in the depth of the mineralized dentine. This finding has been confirmed by the demonstration of oxidative enzyme activity within the odontoblast process. Numerous microtubules and fine filaments are also present in the odontoblast processes, but their function is unknown although it has been suggested that they provide pathways for metabolites.

Microscopic examination of ground sections of dentine reveals the presence of interglobular dentine, most frequently beneath the enamel-dentine junction. These three-dimensional spaces are interpreted as areas of deficient mineralization of the dentine matrix, representing the interstices between calcospherites which have failed to fuse completely. It has been shown, however, that the interstitial spaces visualized in stained decalcified sections are more numerous than the areas of interglobular dentine seen in microradiographs of ground sections. In general the odontoblast processes extend uninterruptedly through the interglobular spaces, although recently it has been suggested that sometimes the tubules themselves expand to become the spaces. Peri-tubular dentine is not found in interglobular spaces. From this it might be argued that mineralized intertubular dentine must be present before peri-tubular dentine is mineralized. However, in some animals peri-tubular dentine forms in the region of the predentine, that is before the intertubular dentine is mineralized. This suggests that the mineralization of dentine may be under the control of the odontoblast processes rather than being a simple physico-chemical reaction of mature dentine matrix. In the absence of this control, not only does intertubular dentine fail to mineralize but neither is peri-tubular dentine formed.

Within the subsurface of the root dentine is the granular layer of Tomes. This is believed to consist of a narrow zone of minute interglobular spaces which may be related to the arcade form of the matrix fibres in this area. Here again, in ground sections, one finds continuity between some of these spaces and the dentine tubules.

Outside Tomes's granular layer a thin structureless hyaline layer can frequently be seen in ground sections. The significance of this layer is not known.

Dentine formation continues slowly throughout life. This later formed dentine may be very difficult to distinguish from the first formed dentine although it can often be recognized by the sudden change in the orientation of the tubules at the interface between the two. This later formed dentine is called 'physiological (or 'regular') secondary dentine'. At one time it was considered that this secondary dentine was formed beneath the cusps of teeth in response to attrition. However, this is unlikely to be true because it is formed in greater amounts at the floor of the pulp chambers in multi-rooted teeth, a position in which such a stimulus does not exist.

REFERENCES

BOYDE, A., and LESTER, K. S. (1966), 'An Electron Microscope Study of Fractured Dentinal Surfaces', *Calc. Tiss. Res.*, **1**, 122.

BRADFORD, E. W. (1967), 'Microanatomy and Histochemistry of Dentine', in *Structural and Chemical Organisation of Teeth* (ed. MILES, A. E. W.). New York: Academic.

FRANK, R. M. (1966), '*Étude au microscopie electronique de l'odontoblasts et du canalicule dentaire humaine*', *Archs oral Biol.*, **11**, 179.

JOHANSEN, E. (1967), 'Ultrastructure of Dentine', in *Structural and Chemical Organisation of Teeth* (ed. MILES, A. E. W.). New York: Academic.

— — and PARKS, H. F. (1962), 'Electron Microscopic Observations on Sound Human Dentine', *Archs oral Biol.*, **7**, 185.

KAYE, H., and HEROLD, R. C. (1966), 'Structure of Human Dentine. I. Phase Contrast, Polarization, Interference and Bright Field Microscopic Observations on the Lateral Branch System', *Ibid.*, **11**, 355.

KRAMER, I. R. H. (1951), 'The Distribution of Collagen Fibrils in the Dentine Matrix', *Br. dent. J.*, **91**, 1.

LESTER, K. S., and BOYDE, A. (1968), 'The Question of von Korff Fibres in Mammalian Dentine', *Calc. Tiss. Res.*, **1**, 273.

PHILLIPAS, G. G. (1961), 'Influence of Occlusal Wear and Age on Formation of Dentine and Size of Pulpchamber', *J. dent. Res.*, **40**, 1186.

— — and APPLEBAUM, E. (1966), 'Age Factor in Secondary Dentine Formation', *Ibid.*, **45**, 778.

SCHMIDT, H. (1961), '*Ein Beitrag zur Morphologie der Interglobularraume im verkalkten Dentin und ihr Nachweis der Entkalkung*', *Archs oral Biol.*, **4**, 63.

SYMONS, N. B. B. (1968), *Dentine and Pulp*. A symposium. Edinburgh: Livingstone.

CHAPTER XIV

DENTINE SENSITIVITY

THE mechanism of dentine sensitivity is one of the most intriguing problems of dental histology and physiology. From common experience, most readers would not dispute that dentine is sensitive. This seems to imply the presence of nerve elements within the dentine, but evidence is accumulating which suggests that the sensory receptors of teeth are located within the pulp. It must also be remembered that histological studies alone cannot explain the mechanism of dentine sensitivity. All these can do is demonstrate a neuro-anatomical pathway associated with dentine sensitivity.

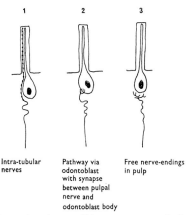

Fig. 49.—Diagram illustrating the possible neuro-anatomical pathways associated with dentine sensitivity.

Three possibilities exist which could explain the sensitivity of dentine. First, that the dentine is indeed innervated; second, that the odontoblast process and cell body have a special sensory function and are connected to a more normal neuro-anatomical pathway starting in the pulp; third, the receptors associated with dentine sensitivity are located within the pulp but are capable of detecting local changes conducted mechanically through the thickness of the dentine (*Fig.* 49). Each of these possibilities will now be discussed in turn, beginning with the evidence for the innervation of dentine.

No dispute exists about the presence of nerve trunks within the pulp. These can readily be demonstrated in several ways. Nor is there much dispute that these nerve trunks spread from the plexus of Raschkow beneath the odontoblasts. The disputed point is whether or not finer nerve elements enter the dentine tubules and run as far as the enamel-dentine junction. Careful and controlled histological studies have shown that nerve-fibres leave the plexus of Raschkow, pass into the predentine as a loop, and pass out again to rejoin the plexus; also, what is more important, nerve-fibres enter the dentine tubules directly (*Fig.* 50). However, the latter observation applies only to a proportion of dentine tubules in any one tooth and this number varies considerably. In some teeth only 1 intratubular fibre per 2000 tubules can be demonstrated. This is the sum of the evidence to suggest that dentine sensitivity is due to nerves within the dentine. Against this hypothesis is the fact that, with one possible exception in the case of the rat incisor, no demonstration has yet been made of intratubular nerve-fibres coursing as far as the enamel-dentine junction. Clinically this junction is reputed to be the most sensitive part of the dentine.

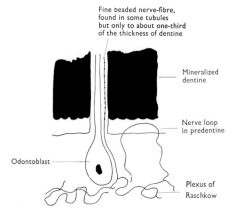

Fig. 50.—Diagrammatic illustration of the location of nerves in dentine.

Logically it might be expected that such a sensitive tissue as dentine would be richly innervated. It may be that the final terminations of the nerve-fibres are beyond the limit of resolution of the optical microscope; also it may be that the silver stains normally used to demonstrate neural elements are too capricious. Not only are silver stains capricious but they also stain reticulin and young collagen fibres which abound in the pulp close to the dentine and which may be confused with nerves. Moreover, demineralized sections are most frequently used in dentine studies and in such sections there will be shrinkage and precipitation of the tubule contents. The precipitated material shows an affinity for silver and can mimic the appearance of fine nerve-fibres. However, there is evidence that in the permanent tooth, the innervation as described above is not established until the tooth has been in function for at least four or five years. Yet the recently erupted tooth is sensitive. There is an alternative explanation for the histological findings outlined above. During the development of the tooth it is known that 'pioneer' nerve-fibres invade the dental papilla at the bell stage of development and that these fibres follow the path of the blood-vessels. However, the ramification of nerves which forms the plexus of Raschkow is not established until root formation is complete. This means that the nerve-fibres must grow towards the dentine if its innervation is to be established. The growing nerve tip approaching the predentine can find itself in one of two situations. It can by chance abut against the opening of the dentine tubule and pass into the lumen of the tubule, between the tubule wall and the odontoblast process. It is easy to conceive that such a growing tip pushes its way along the tubule until it meets the surface of the peri-tubular dentine when its extension ceases (*Fig.* 51). This would explain why intratubular nerve-fibres are only found for a limited distance within the dentine and also why only a proportion of tubules contain them, their distribution depending on

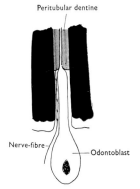

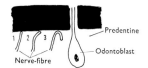

Fig. 52.—Diagram to illustrate three successive steps in the formation of a predentine nerve-loop.

Fig. 51.—Diagram showing how an intratubular nerve-fibre might be restricted by the peri-tubular dentine.

chance. The alternative situation is that a growing nerve-fibre may not enter a dentine tubule but abut against the predentine surface. In this event, the growing tip will retract slightly and readvance at a different angle. A succession of such steps would result in the looping of the nerve-fibre (*Fig.* 52), and such loops could be caught up in the forming dentine.

It is thus fair to say that there is little doubt that mineralized dentine is innervated, but it is another question whether the presence of these few nerve-fibres significantly influences the sensitivity of dentine. The histological demonstration of neural elements in dentine fails to explain the suggested hypersensitivity of the enamel-dentine junction or the sensitivity of newly erupted teeth.

We must now discuss the evidence for considering the odontoblast as a cell capable of transmitting a stimulus in a way that is comparable to a nerve.

Such a hypothesis seems to require, first, that some form of impulse is propagated down an odontoblast, and, second, the presence of a functional connexion between the odontoblasts and those nerve-endings which continue to propagate the impulse. This functional connexion may or may not be a synapse.

In support of this it was at one time reported that acetylcholinesterase was present adjacent to the bodies and processes of the odontoblasts. This enzyme is typically found in association with nerves and its presence in dentine suggested an affinity between nerves and odontoblasts. Second, because odontoblasts are probably of neural crest origin it is not unreasonable to suggest that they may retain the ability of many neural crest cells (e.g., peripheral sensory nerves and postganglionic sympathetic nerves) to propagate an impulse. Third, a recent electron-microscopic study has demonstrated what was described as 'a close functional relationship' (the term 'synapse' was specifically avoided) between nerve-endings and the processes of odontoblasts. Finally, the fact that odontoblast processes branch profusely in the region of the enamel-dentine junction could explain the reported hypersensitivity of the enamel-dentine junction on the basis of a summation phenomenon.

However, all the above findings have been either refuted or disputed. A more reliable method of assessing the presence of acetylcholinesterase has failed to demonstrate its presence in dentine. The membrane potential of odontoblasts has been measured in tissue culture (N.B., not *in vivo*) and found to be too low to take part in an excitable process. Substances known to cause pain when applied to bare nerve-endings do not cause pain when applied to exposed dentine, while substances causing pain when applied to dentine do not cause pain when applied to nerve-endings. These findings all suggest that an odontoblast does not act as a type of nerve. As explained above, the close relationship between nerves and odontoblasts may be due to fortuitous growth rather than evidence of a functional relationship.

If the odontoblast process does not propagate an electrical impulse it remains to explain how a stimulus applied to the largely nerve-free dentine can be transmitted to the nerve-endings deep within the tooth. The possibility exists of a purely physical rather than biological transmission of the stimulus. For example, it has been suggested that temperature changes at the surface of a tooth could be physically transmitted, by conduction, through the mineralized dentine to the pulp. But carefully timed responses to pain-producing stimuli have indicated that the speed of transmission is far greater than could be predicted by simple conduction. The times were closely related to those which could be predicted if the stimulus caused the movement of fluid through the dentine due to surface contractions and expansions consequent on temperature changes.

This is a part of the evidence which suggests that fluid movements in the dentine could be responsible for evoking the initiation of impulses from nerve-endings. It has not been found possible to test this directly; experiments have so far been limited to determining first whether fluid can move through dentine and second whether pain is evoked when the fluid can be presumed to have moved.

The rapid movement of fluid through dentine has now been demonstrated many times *in vitro*. A capillary is sealed to the root of a tooth from which the pulp has been removed (*Fig.* 53). The excavated pulp and the capillary are filled with saline. A cavity is cut into the dentine. If solutions of high osmotic pressure (for instance, sugar solutions) are applied to the cut surface of the dentine, fluid is rapidly sucked through the capillary. Still greater movements are produced by drying the dentine with a blast of air or by cutting the dentine with a drill.

It can be shown that each of the above operations causes pain *in vivo* and that the amount of pain is roughly proportional to the fluid movement observed *in vitro*. It is tentatively concluded that the movement of fluid through dentine causes stimulation of nerve-endings either in the pulp or in the dentine. The fluid which moves may be accommodated in either the periodontoblastic space or the process of the odontoblast, or both. In any event it is probably the eventual movement of interstitial fluid in the pulp which would initiate the stimulation of the nerve fibres. This is the basis of the suggestion that there is a hydrodynamic transmission of pain-producing stimuli.

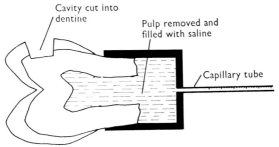

Fig. 53.—Illustrating the method by which movements of fluid through dentine have been measured.

Although the evidence for the concept that pulpal nerves originate the impulse has been summarized briefly here, sufficient has been written to indicate the present trend of opinion concerning dentine sensitivity. Some problems are still outstanding, mainly concerning the extracellular or intracellular nature of the fluid which may move in the dentine tubules. Furthermore, it is not known if the neural elements demonstrated in dentine can be totally excluded from the mechanism of dentine sensitivity.

REFERENCES

ANDERSON, D. J. (1963), *Sensory Mechanisms in Dentine.* Oxford: Pergamon.
— — HANNAM, A. G., and MATHEWS, B. (1970), 'Sensory Mechanisms in Mammalian Teeth and their Supporting Structures', *Physiol. rev.,* **50,** 171.
BRADLAW, R. V. (1936), 'The Innervation of Teeth', *Proc. R. Soc. Med.,* **29,** 507.
BRANNSTROM, M. (1968), 'Physio-pathological Aspects of Dentinal and Pulpal Response to Irritants', in *Dentine and Pulp* (ed. SYMONS, N. B. B.). Edinburgh: Livingstone.
FEARNHEAD, R. W. (1957), 'Histological Evidence for the Innervation of Human Dentine', *J. Anat., Lond.,* **91,** 267.
FRANK, R. M. (1968), 'Relationship between the Odontoblast, its Process and the Nerve Fibre', in *Dentine and Pulp* (ed. SYMONS, N. B. B.). Edinburgh: Livingstone.
POWERS, M. M. (1952), 'The Staining of Nerve Fibres in Teeth', *J. dent Res.,* **31,** 383.
TEN CATE, A. R., and SHELTON, L. (1966), 'Cholinesterase Activity in Human Teeth' *Archs oral Biol.,* **11,** 423.

CHAPTER XV

AMELOGENESIS

ALTHOUGH enamel is ectodermal, as opposed to mesodermal, in origin, and although it contains an extremely high proportion of inorganic salts (96 per cent by weight), its formation displays the same fundamental features found in the other mineralized tissues of the body; a cellular layer produces a matrix which is subsequently mineralized with hydroxyapatite.

At the bell stage of tooth development, when the crown pattern of the tooth is being determined, the base of the enamel organ consists of a single

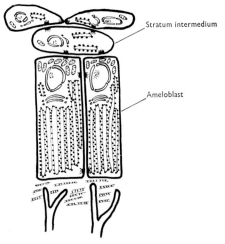

Fig. 54.—The differentiated ameloblast.

layer of short columnar cells, the internal enamel epithelium. The remaining tissues of the enamel organ are the stratum intermedium, stellate reticulum, and external enamel epithelium. At the time of differentiation of the odontoblasts, the cells of the inner enamel epithelium increase in length, their cytoplasm accumulates an increasing amount of 'smooth' and 'rough' endoplasmic reticulum and free ribosomes and their mitochondria move to the end of the cell nearest the stratum intermedium (*Fig.* 54). These changes are of a nature preparatory to the production of enamel; the cell is now termed an 'ameloblast'. The stratum intermedium and the inner enamel epithelium must be regarded as a single functional unit for the production of enamel. Alkaline phosphatase is found exclusively in the stratum intermedium, while the internal enamel epithelium is rich in RNA and has high oxidative enzyme activity. These histochemical features parallel those found in the cells forming other hard tissues.

The point has been made that the formative cells of the other hard tissues differentiate in regions of high vascularity. This is not so in the case of the cells of the internal enamel epithelium. These cells differentiate into functional ameloblasts in a relatively avascular situation. Not until the outer enamel epithelium becomes adjacent to the stratum intermedium with 'collapse' of the stellate reticulum does the former's rich capillary plexus provide the nutritive source for the ameloblasts. Until this vascular supply is established the ameloblasts are rich in glycogen and, because this is lost as the first increments of enamel matrix form, the glycogen could be the source of energy used during the initial period of amelogenesis.

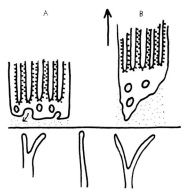

Fig. 55.—A, The initial formation of enamel matrix. B, The formation of a Tomes' process.

With the onset of amelogenesis, the ameloblasts shorten slightly, increase in width, and their cytoplasm comes to contain secretory vacuoles filled with material which under the electron microscope appears stippled. These vacuoles collect at the secretory pole of the cell and by reverse pinocytosis discharge their contents. This discharged material constitutes the organic matrix of the first formed enamel. It is evident, therefore, that enamel is formed by a secretory process and not by a conversion of the protoplasm of the ameloblast as was once believed. The ameloblasts move outwards away from the dentine surface as enamel matrix is secreted. When sufficient matrix has been deposited between the secretory end of an ameloblast and the outer surface of the dentine, the cell membrane of the ameloblast becomes pushed into the matrix as the conical Tomes' process, through which further matrix is secreted (*Fig.* 55). The secretory activity of the ameloblast continues until the full enamel complement is formed.

Apart from knowledge of the proportions of amino-acids there is as yet insufficient reliable knowledge of the structure of the proteins in enamel to present a 'textbook' description. The problem is largely related to the very small quantities of protein present in enamel and the difficulty of isolating it for analysis.

It is possible to demineralize enamel in several different ways to leave a 'soup' containing most of the organic material. There are probably several different proteins in enamel, each having a different solubility in different demineralizing agents. During demineralization some of these proteins may become broken up into large polypeptides, some may remain unbroken. During the subsequent chemical procedures necessary to purify these proteins, other proteins may break up and some of the polypeptides may come together to form polypeptide aggregates of high molecular weight. These 'manufactured' aggregates may then be incorrectly identified as separate proteins. It is therefore very difficult to be certain, following a chemical analysis, that the resultant 'proteins' were in fact present in the original enamel. However, one series of studies has provided convincing evidence that the protein in enamel tufts is quite different from that found in the remainder of the enamel.

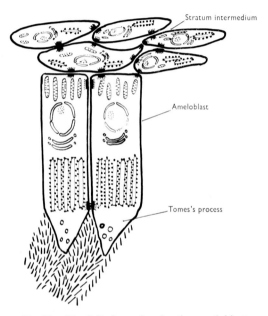

Fig. 56.—The fully formed and active ameloblast.

Valuable information about the proteins can be indirectly obtained from analyses of the amino-acids. Thus it is possible to take the protein 'soup' referred to above, to break all the peptide bonds, and to analyse the proportions of the amino-acids present. The ratios referred to below were derived in this way. By comparing amino-acid analyses of developing and mature enamel it can be shown that large quantities of the amino-acid proline are removed during enamel maturation. This suggests that a protein (or it could be a polypeptide) which is rich in proline is selectively removed from enamel during enamel maturation.

It is thought by some that a keratin-like fibrous protein is present in the enamel matrix. The fibrous nature of this matrix seemed to be proved by the evidence of a complex of interlacing fibres seen with the electron microscope in carefully demineralized sections of enamel. Also various histochemical stains produced the same tinctorial picture in both enamel matrix and keratin. It has already been pointed out that the ultrastructure of the ameloblast does not conform to that of the keratinizing cell (Chapter X). Electron microscopy of developing enamel and X-ray diffraction analyses of the unfixed matrix fail to reveal any evidence of a highly ordered fibre system. The similar staining reactions of enamel matrix and keratin can be explained when it is remembered that the stains employed demonstrate amino-acids and do not give any information as to how the amino-acids are assembled. In fact, biochemical analyses show that the

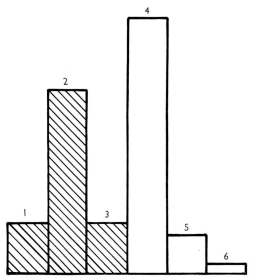

Fig. 57.—Histogram showing the change in amino-acid composition during enamel maturation. Cross hatched = before maturation. The numbers represent the number of amino-acid residues per 1000 total residues. 1, Glycine 67. 2, Proline 243. 3, Histidine 63. 4, Glycine 305. 5, Proline 47. 6, Histidine 9.

ratios of amino-acids in forming enamel matrix are unique. Some salient features are an unusually high content of proline (25 per cent), the presence of the amino-acids histidine, lysine, and arginine in the ratio of 3:1:1, which is not comparable to the 1:4:12 ratio found in eukeratins, and, lastly, the fact that cystine occurs in minimal amounts unlike the keratins which contain at least four times as much of this amino-acid. The large number of proline residues in enamel matrix suggests the presence of a relatively unstable polypeptide. The protein molecules may be incorporated as a concentrated amorphous gel structure, rather than as an orientated assembly of fibres. It is also suggested that this matrix has thixotropic qualities (ability to flow under pressure).

Support for these suggestions is gained from autoradiographic studies of sections of teeth of animals killed at various intervals after injection with labelled amino-acids. These studies demonstrate that although most incorporation of labelled amino-acids takes place rapidly into the newly formed enamel matrix, the labelled material subsequently spreads out, so that after several days all the formed matrix, i.e., matrix formed before and after injection, is labelled. This means that the proteins of the enamel matrix in which the amino-acids have been incorporated are labile. Within this distinctive matrix growth of apatite crystals occurs. The introduction of mineral salts occurs after the formation of a layer of enamel matrix about 500 Å thick. The initial epitactic foci may be the adjacent dentine hydroxyapatite. The hydroxyapatite is in the form of tape-like crystallites, which, when they are first seen in the electron microscope, are thin and relatively widely separated within the matrix (*Fig.* 56). The crystallites thicken rapidly by addition to their sides and it is thought that the intervening matrix is squeezed out from between them in the direction of the ameloblasts where it is possible that it is utilized once more to initiate further nuclei of crystallization.

A Formative

B Resorptive

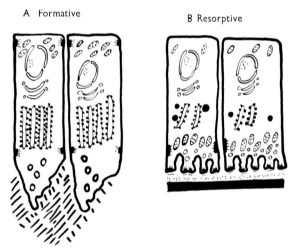

Fig. 58.—Diagram illustrating the differences between the ameloblast at the formative and at the resorptive stage.

Enamel is exceedingly highly mineralized and during its formation qualitative and quantitative changes take place within the enamel matrix to accommodate the increased mineral matter. For many years it was thought that enamel formation occurred in two separate phases: an initial phase involving the deposition of a partially mineralized matrix and, when the entire thickness of enamel matrix had been laid down, a second phase of enamel maturation whereby the final high mineral content of enamel was obtained. This latter process was supposed to occur from the outer surface of the enamel and progress inwards towards the enamel dentine junction. It is now known from microradiographic studies that mineralization of enamel is more of a continuous phenomenon which lags behind the deposition of the matrix. Even so, as the final high mineralization of enamel is attained a fairly rapid change occurs in the nature of the organic matrix. There is a loss of water and amino-acids, especially histidine and proline, so that the final matrix of enamel not only has less protein but has a different composition from that initially secreted by the ameloblasts (*Fig.* 57). How these changes are brought about is not certain but more and more evidence is accumulating which implicates the ameloblast. At the final stages of removal of organic material the ameloblast shows certain chemical and ultrastructural changes which suggest an absorptive function. In the rodent there is an increase in surface area of the cell adjacent to the formed enamel and an accumulation of mitochondria in this region. Numerous vesicles are found, indicating uptake

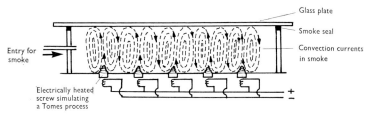

Fig. 59.—Diagrammatic section of the smoke chamber.

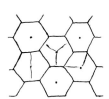

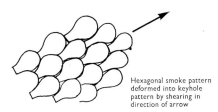

Fig. 60.—Pattern seen in the smoke when viewed from above through the glass plate.

Fig. 61.—Deformation of smoke pattern by moving glass plate in direction of the arrow.

of material, and the Golgi apparatus becomes well developed and has been associated with lysosome development (*Fig.* 58). Hydrolytic and oxidative enzyme activity increase dramatically and amino-peptidase activity becomes demonstrable. This latter enzyme is also found in areas of bone resorption. Comparable information is not yet available in primates but the reduced ameloblasts in monkey material have been shown to contain many vacuoles suggestive of uptake of extracellular material.

It will become clear in the next chapter that a sudden change of crystallite orientation is responsible for the prism outline seen with the electron microscope. The factors determining the orientation of crystallites are not known precisely. Recently, however, it has been proposed that the crystallites become orientated along lines of flow developed within secreted enamel matrix.

Two artificial systems have been designed to demonstrate this contention. The first is a smoke chamber in which convection currents are established in the smoke to mimic flow lines (*Fig.* 59). When these are observed through the glass plate forming the top of the smoke chamber

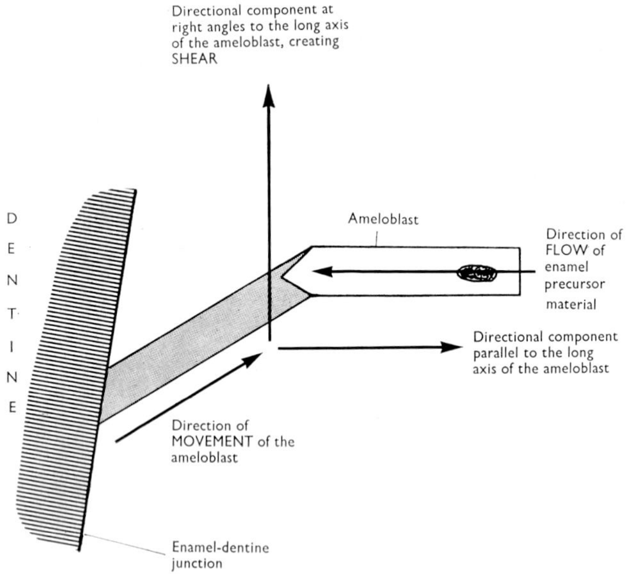

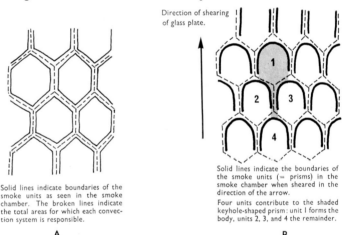

Directional component at right angles to the long axis of the ameloblast, creating SHEAR

D E N T I N E

Ameloblast

Direction of FLOW of enamel precursor material

Directional component parallel to the long axis of the ameloblast

Direction of MOVEMENT of the ameloblast

Enamel-dentine junction

Fig. 62.—The direction of movement of an ameloblast can be resolved into two components, one at right angles to the long axis of the ameloblast and one parallel to the long axis. It can be seen that the former produces the shear.

Direction of shearing of glass plate.

Solid lines indicate boundaries of the smoke units as seen in the smoke chamber. The broken lines indicate the total areas for which each convection system is responsible.

Solid lines indicate the boundaries of the smoke units (= prisms) in the smoke chamber when sheared in the direction of the arrow.

Four units contribute to the shaded keyhole-shaped prism: unit 1 forms the body, units 2, 3, and 4 the remainder.

A

B

Fig. 63.—Details of smoke patterns as seen from above, A, without shearing, B, when sheared.

hexagonal patterns are seen which are similar to the cross-sectional appearance of the ameloblasts (*Fig.* 60). If the glass plate is sheared, the hexagonal smoke patterns convert to a keyhole-shape resembling the cross-sectional appearance of human enamel prism (*Fig.* 61). By moving the glass plate in different directions, smoke patterns conforming to the cross-sectional appearance of prisms of other types of mammalian enamel can be produced.

The second artificial system involves the use of iron filings and magnets. When magnets are drawn under a card sprinkled with iron filings, the filings arrange themselves along the lines of magnetic force. If the magnets are moved in a skewed manner so that a shearing component is introduced,

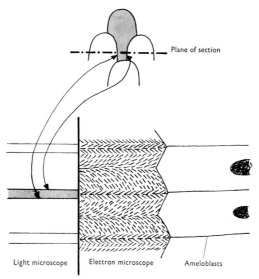

Fig. 64.—Diagrammatic representation of the probable appearance of amelogenesis as it would appear in a transverse section of the tooth. Where neighbouring ameloblasts touch, two changes in crystallite orientation can be seen in the electron micrograph. The same area is seen in the light microscope as a zone of interprismatic substance (left) which is in reality part of a prism out of the plane of section.

the iron filings become orientated in such a way as to mimic the crystallite orientation seen in longitudinal sections of enamel. The results obtained from these two artificial systems suggest that the crystallites in enamel are orientated along lines of flow generated within the enamel matrix as it is secreted from the ameloblasts. The shearing factor is generated in human amelogenesis by virtue of the angulation of the ameloblast to the forming enamel front (*Fig.* 62).

It used to be thought that one ameloblast was responsible for one prism. However, reference to *Fig.* 63 substantiates the electron microscopic findings that four ameloblasts are responsible for each keyhole-shaped prism. Two diagrams of the electron microscopic appearance of amelogenesis are shown in *Figs.* 64 and 65. One represents a transverse section of the tooth and the other a longitudinal section of the tooth. In studying these diagrams it must be remembered that the prism borders seen under the light microscope are related to sudden changes in crystallite orientation. It can be seen in *Fig.* 64 that two sudden changes of orientation can be related to adjacent ameloblasts in the transverse plane of the tooth, whereas only one change, related to the tip of each Tomes' process, can be seen in the longitudinal plane of the tooth (*Fig.* 65).

Thus three theories have been proposed to explain the orientation of the crystallites. First, the crystallites grow at right angles to the surfaces of the Tomes' process; second, they grow at right angles to the mineralizing front, but that this orientation is modified by a 'stroking' factor due to the

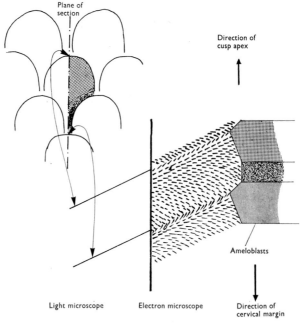

Fig. 65.—Diagrammatic representation of the appearance of amelogenesis as it would appear in the longitudinal section of the tooth. The electron micrograph shows a single change in crystallite orientation related to the tip of the Tomes' process. The shading shows the contribution of each ameloblast to the enamel prism. Lack of a Tomes' process on the central ameloblast is due to the plane of section which misses this process but passes through the process of adjacent ameloblasts.

angulation of the long axis of the ameloblasts to their direction of movement in the longitudinal plane of the tooth; third, they are orientated along flow lines produced in the enamel precursor material by the flow of secreted material from the ameloblasts.

At the completion of amelogenesis the ameloblasts secrete a layer of organic material about 1 μ thick over the completed enamel surface. This layer is the primary enamel cuticle (Chapter XXII) and after this structure has been formed the ameloblasts, together with the remaining tissues of the dental organ, form Nasmyth's membrane, which is involved in the eruptive sequence and the formation of the epithelial attachment.

REFERENCES

BOYDE, A. (1965), 'The Structure of Developing Mammalian Dental Enamel', in *Tooth Enamel* (ed., STACK, M. V., and FEARNHEAD, R. W.). Bristol: Wright.
BURGESS, R. C., and MACLAREN C. M. (1965), 'Proteins in Developing Bovine Enamel', in *Tooth Enamel* (ed. STACK, M. V., and FEARNHEAD, R. W.). Bristol: Wright.
CRABB, H. S. M., and DARLING, A. I. (1962), *The Pattern of Progressive Mineralization in Human Dental Enamel.* Oxford: Pergamon.
EASTOE, J. E. (1963), 'The Amino-Acid Composition of Proteins in Dentine and Enamel from Developing Human Deciduous Teeth', *Archs oral Biol.*, **8,** 633.
KALLENBACH, E. (1968), 'Fine Structure of Rat Incisor Ameloblasts during Enamel Maturation', *J. ultrastruct. Res.*, **22,** 90.
NYLEN, M. U., EAMES, E. D., and OMNELL, K. A. (1963), 'Crystal Growth in Rat Enamel', *J. cell. Biol.*, **18,** 109.
OSBORN, J. W. (1970), 'The Mechanism of Prism Formation in Teeth: a Hypothesis', *Calc. Tiss., Res.*, **5,** 115.
— — (1970), 'The Mechanism of Ameloblast Movement: a Hypothesis', *Ibid.*, **5,** 344.
REITH, E. J. (1970), 'The Stages of Amelogenesis as observed in Molar Teeth of Young Rats', *J. ultrastruct. Res.*, **30,** 111.
RONNHOLM, E. (1962a), 'The Amelogenesis of Human Teeth as revealed by Electron Microscopy. II, The Development of Enamel Crystallites', *Ibid.*, **6,** 249.
— — (1962b), 'An Electron Microscopic Study of Amelogenesis in Human Teeth. I, The Fine Structure of Ameloblasts,' *Ibid.*, **6,** 299.
STACK, M. V., and FEARNHEAD, R. W., ed. (1965), *Tooth Enamel.* Bristol: Wright.
YOUNG, R. W., and GREULICH, R. C. (1963), 'Distinctive Autoradiographic Patterns of Glycine Incorporation in Rat Enamel and Dentine Matrices', *Archs oral Biol.*, **8,** 509.

CHAPTER XVI

ENAMEL STRUCTURE

LIGHT microscopists had described all the known structures in human enamel, including the crystallites and their orientation (which had been inferred from polarization microscopy and X-ray diffraction studies), before the tissue was thoroughly investigated by electron microscopists. It is convenient to start with their observations because many of the structures they have described have yet to be seen by electron microscopists.

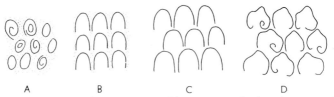

A   B   C   D

Fig. 66.—Illustrating the appearances of human enamel prisms in cross-section: A, Close to the enamel dentine junction; B, At about 50μ from the enamel-dentine junction; C, Within most of the enamel; D, In some regions at the surface of the enamel. Generally agreed interprismatic regions are stippled.

To the light microscopists the unit of enamel is the prism. It seems probable that most prisms extend through the full thickness of the enamel, widening from a diameter of about 3μ near the enamel-dentine junction to about 6μ at the surface of the tooth. This widening is accounted for by the fact that near the enamel-dentine junction prisms are separated by larger interprismatic regions and also that the inner surface of the enamel has a smaller area than the outer surface. Recent evidence suggests that some prisms fail to reach the surface of the tooth from which it can be concluded that some ameloblasts die before the full thickness of enamel is deposited.

Near the enamel-dentine junction, in true cross-section, human prisms may have any of the appearances shown in *Fig.* 66A. They are widely separated by an interprismatic region. At about 50μ from the enamel-dentine junction they have enlarged considerably at the expense of the interprismatic region and are arranged as in *Fig.* 66B. At about 100μ from the enamel-dentine junction they have the appearance shown in *Fig.* 66C and continue to appear like this until very close to the surface of the tooth where they may again become very irregular (*Fig.* 66D) or their borders may disappear.

Within the last few years it has become fashionable to describe human enamel as consisting of 'keyhole-shaped' prisms (shaded in *Fig.* 67B), locked together in such a way that there is no interprismatic region. Previously the structure shown in *Fig.* 67A was described as consisting of roughly hexagonal or circular prisms separated by interprismatic 'substance', a material which was thought to be less mineralized than the body of the prism (*Fig.* 67C). However, because electron microscopists have concluded that this latter 'substance' contains identical proportions of hydroxyapatite to that of the prism bodies it is preferable to use the term interprismatic 'region'. It will be observed from the diagram that the two conflicting descriptions of human enamel structure (keyhole-shaped prisms without interprismatic regions and circular prisms separated by interprismatic regions) are related solely to differences in terminology. There is no disagreement about the structure being described (*Fig.* 67A).

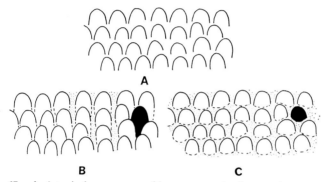

Fig. 67.—A, A typical appearance of human enamel prisms cut in cross-section. One terminology refers to the majority of these prisms as being 'keyhole-shaped' (black prism in B) and recognizes interprismatic regions only where they are stippled in this diagram. The other terminology (C) refers to prisms as 'roughly circular' (black) and to the remaining region as being 'interprismatic'.

Both interpretations require the construction of imaginary lines in order to complete the prism border. Because there is general agreement that all other forms of prismatic enamel contain interprismatic regions it seems to us that it is less confusing, more consistent, and probably more realistic to describe human enamel prisms as roughly circular, bearing in mind that the prism body is in continuity with the interprismatic region cervically.

Prisms bend from side to side in the transverse plane of the tooth but are approximately straight in the vertical plane of the tooth (*Fig.* 68). A horizontal row of prisms all follow a similar path which is slightly out of phase with the paths of prisms in adjacent rows. This phase difference produces the sinuous structure shown on the left of *Fig.* 68. The borders of prisms reflect a small quantity of incident light. It can be seen that if incident light is reflected from the surface of a longitudinal section of enamel the shaded regions in *Fig.* 68 would not reflect light up the microscope and would therefore appear dark. The unshaded regions would appear bright, because they reflect light up the microscope. This banded appearance is an epiphenomenon known as the 'Hunter-Schreger bands'. By changing the direction of the light the brightness of the bands is reversed. Towards the outer one-third of the enamel the prisms all pass straight to the surface and it is evident that it will no longer be possible to see bands.

As a first approximation it is helpful to think of human enamel as consisting of a series of single-prism thick, coaxial, hollow cones with open apices lying against the enamel-dentine junction and their free edges at the surface of the tooth (*Fig.* 69). Each cone is a single layer of undulating tapered prisms. The phase difference between the bends of prisms contained in adjacent cones has been described above. At the tip of the cusp the apical angles of the cones are so acute that most longitudinal sections of a tooth cut the faces of several cones and the phase differences

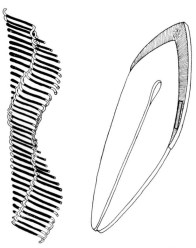

Fig. 68.—A ground section of a tooth is represented on the right. Prisms from the boxed region are represented on the left.

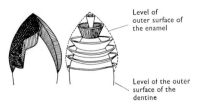

Fig. 69.—Block diagrams illustrating the structure of enamel.

between the undulating prisms contained in each of the cones are superimposed on each other. The resultant apparent intertwining of prisms produces a gnarled appearance (gnarled enamel) which obscures a regularity of structure which can only be observed in transverse sections of the tooth taken through the cuspal enamel.

Contrary to previous descriptions, prisms in the cervical region of permanent teeth are not directed outwards and cervically but are generally approximately horizontal.

Three-dimensional reconstructions of enamel prisms reveal that many undulate at intervals of about 4μ–6μ (*Fig.* 70). Previous studies of prisms seen in two dimensions suggested that these undulations were varicosities and constrictions. It has been speculated that these irregularities may correspond with the cross-striations of the prisms. This does not conflict with the speculation that the cross-striations may result from regular variations in the inorganic/organic ratio of substances along the length of the prism produced in response to a diurnal variation in the 4μ per day rate of enamel formation.

To the light microscopist the prism sheath appears to be about 0·5μ wide. Apart from their observations on the structure of the interprismatic

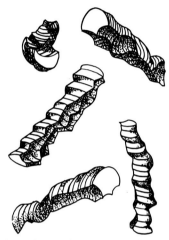

Fig. 70.—Drawings of wax-plate reconstructions of enamel prisms.

region, the other major contribution to an understanding of the morphology of enamel which has been contributed by electron microscopy is that the prism sheath is at most about 0·1μ wide. Indeed, many electron microscopists consider that a sheath *per se* does not exist and that a prism is bounded solely by an interface between crystallites of different orientation. However, a close study of electron micrographs which have been considered to demonstrate this interface seems always to reveal an irregular crystallite-free region (a region of microporosity) where the cervical ends of the crystallites in the more cuspal prism unevenly abut against the sides of the crystallites in the cervically adjacent prism (*Fig.* 71). Without the presence of this crystallite-free region (which being unmineralized, has a refractive index quite different from that of the crystallites) it is difficult to explain why the sides of prisms reflect or scatter light in such a way that the sheath appears about 0·5μ wide to the light microscopist. It has recently been shown that crystallites of the sheath differ from those of the prism.

Within approximately 12μ of the surface of the enamel, in many regions the crystallites are all parallel to the long axes of the prisms and the irregular, microporous, crystallite-free prism sheath no longer exists. The enamel in these regions therefore appears structureless to the light microscopist. The parallel arrangement (and therefore closer packing) of the crystallites and the absence of prism sheaths probably accounts for the observation that the surface enamel is the most highly mineralized.

When sections of enamel are placed in aqueous solutions of certain substances some of the solution diffuses into the enamel and changes its optical properties, particularly the degree of birefringence. The change in birefringence can be measured and is related to the refractive index of the aqueous solution and the amount that diffuses into the enamel. Since the refractive index of the solution is known the amount that has diffused into the enamel can be calculated. It is found that the size of the molecules of the dissolved substance determines the amount which can penetrate into the spaces in the enamel and it is assumed that the volume diffusing when the solution of smallest molecular size is used represents the volume of spaces present in enamel. In this way it can be shown that enamel contains a system of micropores which act as a molecular sieve and that the volume of pores is about 0·2 per cent of the enamel volume. Attempts have been made to show that the optical properties of the striae of Retzius and the cross-striations are related to differences in the amount of pores present in them as compared with the rest of the enamel.

Fig. 71.—Typical appearance of the border between two longitudinally sectioned prisms. There is a region of microporosity between the cervical border of the more cuspal prism and the cuspal border of the more cervical prism.

The brown striae of Retzius seem to reflect a further phasic nature of enamel formation. The cross-striations are probably related to daily increments whereas the striae appear to be 4 day to 16 day increments.

It is generally supposed that, like the cross-striations, the striae are formed in relation to some systemic influence. Two features support this contention. First, neonatal lines seem to be well marked striae. Second, it has sometimes been observed that, taking into account the times at which they have been formed, the striae in all the teeth of a dentition are the same. In other words, the supposed systemic stimulus affected all developing teeth at the same time. However, so far the evidence for this latter conclusion seems limited. In many sections of enamel, striae are invisible because they are oblique to the plane of section; they can usually be seen if the section is tilted under the microscope.

It is a simple enough matter to observe brown striae but it has been found very difficult to give a uniform description of them. They may be between 150μ thick down to the thickness of a cross-striation, they may be hypo- or hypermineralized, they may be continuous or discontinuous, and clear striae, as opposed to brown, have also been described. The borders of prisms within the thicker brown striae are particularly optically dense and it may be that the brown colour is due to blue light (short wavelength) being abnormally scattered at these borders. This is supported by the observation that striae are blue-white when seen by reflected light. It has been speculated without evidence that within striae crystallites may be larger or smaller and that they may be orientated differently from crystallites in adjacent regions (similar speculations have been made on enamel structure in the region of the cross-striations).

It has been reported that in association with striae prisms may bend cervically or that they may bend in the transverse plane of the tooth.

A series of fine furrows can be seen surrounding the surface of young teeth. These are called 'perikymata'. Ground longitudinal sections of teeth show that the brown striae meet the enamel surface at these furrows. From this relationship it is suggested that, during amelogenesis, a certain number of ameloblasts cease secreting at the same time. The series of ameloblasts immediately basal to these continue to secrete and the repetition of this cycle produces the system of perikymata, visible as a

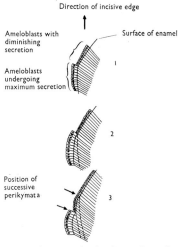

Fig. 72.—Diagrams of successive steps in the formation of perikymata, also showing their relationships to the brown striae of Retzius (broken lines).

regular series of furrows in the outline of the enamel on the section (*Fig.* 72). The scanning electron microscope has shown that in the base of the furrows prism outlines can be distinguished again suggesting early cessation of amelogenesis by groups of prisms.

Three further features of enamel can be seen in ground sections. Enamel lamellae are irregular vertical sheets of organic or hypomineralized matrix extending from the tooth surface often as far as, and occasionally beyond, the enamel-dentine junction. It has been suggested that they develop along planes of tension within the developing enamel, a slight disturbance leading to a failure of mineralization along the plane. Some of these lamellae may open up during development and cells from the dental organ collect in the cleft. Finally, with advancing age, a third type of lamella may form in which the underlying dentine tends to contract so that the enamel, now unsupported, fractures. Organic material from the oral cavity will then collect in the split.

Groups of ribbon-like structures extend from the enamel-dentine junction into the enamel for up to one-third of its thickness. These constitute the 'enamel tufts', so called on account of their resemblance, when seen in transverse ground sections of teeth, to tufts of grass. A reconstruction of a small part of a tuft is shown in *Fig*. 73. Each tuft consists of a number of disconnected 'leaves' which appear to coincide with thickenings of the prism sheaths. In a recent study it was pointed out that when a substance changes from the liquid to the solid state contractions occur. In enamel, hydroxyapatite changes from the ionic (liquid)

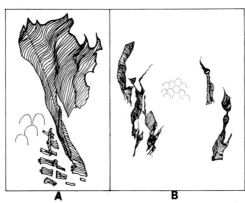

A   **B**

Fig. 73.—Reconstructions of tufts in enamel. The enamel cusp is towards the top and the cervical margin towards the bottom. The prisms outlines indicated in each reconstruction are about 5µ wide.

state in the ameloblast secretions to the solid state in the enamel crystallites. With the change of state, contractions will be expected and it is possible that these contractions could lead to the widening of prism sheaths which corresponds with the tufts. Evidently the tufts will follow the direction of prisms. At the same time it was suggested that the microporosity corresponding with prism sheaths themselves may also be caused by similar contractions. Microradiographic techniques show these regions to be hypocalcified, while diffusion experiments show them to be more permeable.

Frequently one can find in ground sections evidence of the continuation of odontoblast processes across the enamel-dentine junction into the enamel. These constitute the enamel spindles and they are to be found beneath the tips of cusps. The spindles lie parallel to the long axes of the ameloblasts at the start of amelogenesis and they become partly mineralized along with the developing enamel.

REFERENCES

BOYDE, A. (1969), 'Electron Microscopic Observations relating to the Nature and Development of Prism Decussation in Mammalian Dental Enamel', *Bull. Grpmt int. Rech. scient. Stomat.* **12**, 151.

FOSSE, G. (1964), 'The Number of Prism Bases on the Inner and Outer Surface of the Enamel Mantle of Human Teeth', *J. dent. Res.*, **43**, 57.

FOSSE, G. (1968), 'A Quantitative Analysis of the Numerical Density and the Distributional Pattern of Prisms and Ameloblasts in Dental Enamel and Tooth Germs', *Acta odont. scand.*, **26**, 573.

FUJITA, T. (1939), '*Uber die Retzius'schen Parallelstreifen des Zahnschmelzes*', *Anat. Anz.*, **86**, 350.

GLAS, J. E., and NYLEN, M. U. (1965), 'A Correlated Electron Microscopical and Microradiographic Study of Human Enamel', *Archs oral Biol.*, **10**, 893.

GUSTAFSON, A. (1959), 'A Morphologic Investigation of Certain Variations in the Structure and Mineralization of Human Dental Enamel', *Odont. Tidskr.*, **67**, 361.

GUSTAFSON, G., and GUSTAFSON, A. (1967), 'Microanatomy and Histochemistry of Enamel', in *Structural and Chemical Organisation of Teeth*, (ed. MILES, A. E. W.), vol. 2. New York: Academic.

GUSTAVSEN, F., and SILNESS, J. (1969), 'Crystal Shape in the Prism Sheath Region of Sound Human Enamel', *Acta odont. scand.*, **27**, 617.

HELMCKE, J.-G. (1967), 'Ultrastructure of Enamel', in *Structural and Chemical Organisation of Teeth* (ed. MILES, A. E. W.). New York: Academic.

HEUSER, H. (1961), '*Die structur des menslichen zahnschmelzes in oberfläch en histologischen bild (replica technik)*', *Archs oral Biol.*, **4**, 50.

JOHNSON, N. W. (1967), 'Some Aspects of the Ultrastructure of Early Human Enamel Caries seen with the Electron Microscope', *Ibid.*, **12**, 1505.

MECKEL, A. H., GRIEBSTEIN, W. J., and NEAL, R. J. (1965), 'Structure of Mature Human Dental Enamel as observed by Electronmicroscopy', *Ibid.*, **10**, 775.

OSBORN, J. W. (1965), 'The Nature of the Hunter-Schreger Bands in Enamel', *Ibid.*, **10**, 929.

— — (1967), '3-dimensional Reconstructions of Enamel Prisms', *J. dent. Res.*, **46**, 1412.

— — (1968a), 'Directions and Inter-relationships of Enamel Prisms from the Sides of Human Teeth', *Ibid.*, **47**, 217.

— — (1968b), 'Directions and Inter-relationship of Prisms in Cuspal and Cervical Enamel of Human Teeth', *Ibid.*, **47**, 395.

— — (1968c), 'The Cross-sectional Outlines of Human Enamel Prisms', *Acta anat.*, **70**, 493.

— — (1969), 'The 3-dimensional Morphology of the Tufts in Human Enamel', *Ibid.*, **73**, 481.

— — (1971), 'A Relationship between the Striae of Retzius and Prism Directions in the Transverse Plane of the Tooth', *Archs oral Biol.*, in the press.

POOLE, D. F. G., and BROOKS, A. W. (1961), 'The Arrangement of Crystallites in Enamel Prisms', *Ibid.*, **5**, 14.

RIPA, L. W., GWINNETT, A. J., and BUONOCORE, M. G. (1965), 'The Prismless Outer Layer of Deciduous and Permanent Enamel', *Ibid.*, **11**, 41.

SCHOUR, I., and HOFFMAN, M. M. (1939), 'Studies in Tooth Development II. The Rate of Apposition of Enamel and Dentine in Man and other Mammals', *J. dent. Res.*, **18**, 161.

STACK, M. V., and FEARNHEAD, R. W., ed. (1965), *Tooth Enamel*. Bristol: Wright.

CHAPTER XVII

CEMENTOGENESIS

CEMENTOGENESIS begins shortly after the fragmentation of Hertwig's root sheath. Fragmentation of the root sheath permits penetration of the connective tissue cells of the follicle so that they come to lie between the remnants of the root sheath and the thin shell of newly formed dentine. In addition it has recently been shown that these cells migrate apically from the zone of disruption of the root sheath so that connective tissue cells come to lie between the newly formed dentine and the intact root sheath.

These ectomesenchymal cells (*see* Chapter XIX) of the follicle then differentiate into cement-forming cells or cementoblasts. The cells are characterized by the presence of numerous mitochondria, a great deal of rough surfaced endoplasmic reticulum, and a prominent Golgi complex. Histochemically they have a high hydrolytic and oxidative enzyme content. There is evidence that at the time of disruption of Hertwig's sheath, there is a local increase in the number of collagen fibres of the follicle, so that the connective tissue which ultimately intervenes between the root sheath and the dentine is predominantly fibrous. The factors responsible for cementoblast differentiation and for the increased fibrillogenesis are unknown.

The fibrous connective tissue in contact with the root dentine contributes to the first formed cement matrix. It would appear, however, that additional collagen fibres and ground substance are contributed as a result of cementoblast activity to form the definitive unmineralized cement matrix or cementoid. The fibres of this matrix appear to show no preferred orientation. The formation of cement matrix has therefore many parallels with the formation of the dentine matrix in that in both cases there is a dual origin of fibres and of ground substance. When sufficient organic matrix has been formed it becomes mineralized by the deposition within it of hydroxyapatite in the form of either plates or spicules. The manner in which the hydroxyapatite is deposited within the cement matrix has recently been investigated and found to occur as follows. They form at the dentine cement interface, growing from the crystals of the dentine into, onto, and between the collagenous fibrils of the cement matrix.

As matrix formation proceeds, the cement-forming cells can be incorporated within the developing cement where they become cementocytes, or they may remain on the surface of the forming cement as more rounded cells lacking processes. Two types of cement are thus recognized, cellular and acellular respectively. Cementocytes are characterized by processes radiating towards the periodontal ligament and their cytoplasm shows a drastic reduction in the number of organelles when compared to the cementoblast.

Cement is the tissue whereby the fibres of the periodontal ligament gain attachment to the root of the tooth. Before the tooth erupts the fibres of the tooth follicle become incorporated in the cement matrix. These original fibres are arranged approximately parallel to the root surface. After eruption of the tooth, however, the fibres of the periodontal ligament lie oblique to the root surface and it is obvious that they must be incorporated within the cement, otherwise no attachment would be made. These principal fibres of the periodontal ligament are large, rope-like bundles of collagen fibres which, as they approach the cement, untwine to form smaller fibre bundles. It is these smaller fibre bundles which enter the cementoid where their termination is as yet undetermined. Until recently it was thought that the fibres entering the cement (Sharpey's fibres) remained non-mineralized in the surface layers, and became mineralized deeper within this hard tissue. Electron microscopic evidence, however, suggests that these fibres become mineralized as soon as they enter the cement. However, it seems that there is a differential mineralization in that the hydroxyapatite associated with the collagen of Sharpey fibres lies on the surface of the collagen whereas the cement collagen has hydroxyapatite within the macromolecules.

It has been suggested that cementogenesis represents a gradual mineralization of the periodontal ligament. On the other hand, it can be argued that the periodontal ligament and the cement are different, but closely related, tissues both derived from the same source, the dental follicle, and both being specialized forms of connective tissue.

In general there is a direct relationship between the thickness of cement and the age of the tooth. However, its growth is most rapid in the apical regions where it is formed to compensate for active eruption of the tooth which itself compensates for occlusal wear. The phasic nature of its deposition results in incremental lines which have been described as hyper- or hypomineralized. No explanation has been offered for the presence of hypermineralized lines but the hypomineralized lines are comparable to the resting lines present in bone.

On the surface of the root dentine in premolars and molars a variety of cement characterized by wide irregular branching spaces is frequently found. This is the intermediate cement. There is diagreement as to the origin of the cells that at one time occupied these spaces. It has been suggested that these spaces once contained epithelial cells derived from Hertwig's root sheath that had become trapped on the dentine surface during the formation of the first layers of dentine. Alternatively, that during eruption of the cheek teeth, cementocytes whose processes have become attached to the cement and whose periodontal surface is attached to the connective tissue become pulled upwards and distorted by movement of the erupting tooth. A further opinion asserts that the lacunae in this type of cement are occupied by odontoblasts which are trapped on the outer surface of the dentine at the start of dentinogenesis, subsequently being engulfed by the forming cement. The many interpretations of intermediate cement may be the result of species differences. It has recently been shown that in the rodent epithelial root-sheath cells do become trapped in first formed cement. However, several studies on cementogenesis provide no evidence of entrapment of root-sheath cells in man. On the other hand human intermediate cement has been shown to contain cells, larger than cementocytes, which are surrounded by un-mineralized areas. The origin of these cells remains speculative but it seems that a root sheath origin can be excluded.

REFERENCES

BERNARD, G. W. (1970), 'Initial Calcification of Cementum'. Abstract of a paper given at the 48th meeting of the International Association for Dental Research. Supplement to *J. dent. Res.*

FURSETH, R. (1969), 'The Five Structures of the Cellular Cementum of Young Human Teeth', *Archs oral Biol.*, **14**, 1147.

LESTER, K. (1969), 'The Incorporation of Epithelial Cells by Cementum', *J. ultrastruct. Res.*, **27**, 63.

LISTGARTEN, M. A. (1970), 'Ultrastructure of Cementogenesis in Human Teeth'. Abstract of a paper given at the 48th meeting of the International Association for Dental Research. Supplement to *J. dent. Res.*

SELVIG, K. A. (1964), 'Ultrastructural Study of Cementum Formation', *Acta odont. scand.*, **22**, 105.

CHAPTER XVIII

ROOT FORMATION

IT will be recalled from Chapter III that the outer and inner enamel epithelia are continuous at the cervical edge of the enamel organ, forming the cervical loop. In the late bell stage of development, when apposition of the hard tissues of the crown is well advanced, the cervical loop grows to form a double layer of epithelial cells known as 'Hertwig's root sheath'.

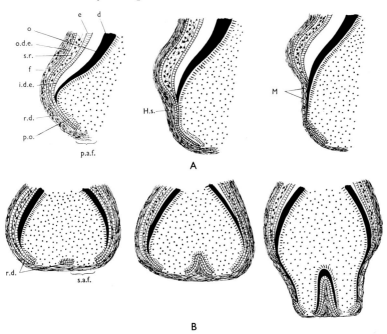

Fig. 74.—Diagrams of three successive stages in root formation, A, in a single-rooted tooth, B, in a two-rooted tooth. Not to scale. d, dentine; e, enamel; f, tooth follicle; H.s., Hertwig's root sheath; i.d.e., inner dental epithelium; M, Malassez rests; o, odontoblasts; o.d.e., outer dental epithelium; p.a.f., primary apical foramen; p.o., differentiating odontoblasts; r.d, epithelial root diaphragm; s.a.f., secondary apical foramen; s.r., stellate reticulum. In A there is a single persistent primary apical foramen. In B the primary apical foramen is rapidly divided to produce two secondary apical foramina.

It is under the influence of this sheath that the roots develop. Frequently one finds in histological sections a few stellate cells sandwiched between the inner and outer epithelia in the root sheath. During development, Hertwig's sheath grows basally between the tooth follicle and the dental papilla and it comes to enclose the papilla except for an opening at its base, known as the 'primary apical foramen' (*Fig.* 74). Hence, root morphogenesis is bound up with the dynamic activity of Hertwig's sheath.

At first Hertwig's sheath is angled beneath the dental papilla in which form it has been termed a 'root diaphragm'. It seems likely that the base of the growing dental papilla pushes the root sheath outwards moulding it to the shape of the base of the fibrous follicle. As the major cusps form on the crown of a molariform tooth, the papilla pushes irregularly outwards as a number of lobes. These lobes produce corresponding 'bays' in the outline of the root diaphragm which surrounds it. The 'bays' correspond

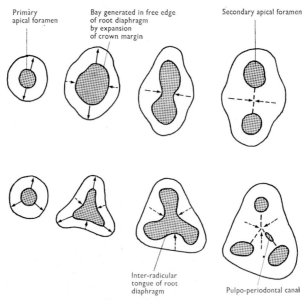

Fig. 75.—Diagrams showing successive stages in the process of subdivision of the primary apical foramen, as seen from below, producing a two- and a three-rooted tooth. The shaded area represents the papilla seen through the apical foramen. The solid arrows show the direction of expansion of the crown margin. The broken arrows show the direction of growth of the inter-radicular tissue tongues of the root diaphragm. Not to scale.

in number and location with the definitive roots (*Fig.* 75). The tongues of epithelial tissue separating the bays now grow inwards to outline the secondary apical foramina and to fuse near the centre of the crown base: the number of the roots thus corresponds with the number of bays in the root diaphragm. The fact that the outward expansion of the papilla generates bays in the root diaphragm might create the impression that there is no intrinsic growth in the diaphragm. However, although not as abundant as might be expected, mitosis figures are found in the cells of the diaphragm from its inception indicating its growth in area. This growth is masked because the base of the dental papilla is expanding at the same rate as the root diaphragm is growing to surround it. Only in regions where the rate of diaphragm growth is greater than the rate of expansion of the base of the dental papilla can the diaphragm divide the root base into separate root areas.

Each secondary apical foramen will ultimately open at a root apex. Where the tongues of tissue meet, running from near the centre of the crown base to the inner aspect of each root, junction lines form, which may be visible as low dentine ridges on the completed tooth. Local defects may occur along these junction lines to produce pulpo-periodontal canals each containing a blood-vessel and a nerve. These are found most commonly in the root bifurcations of deciduous molars. If the adjacent

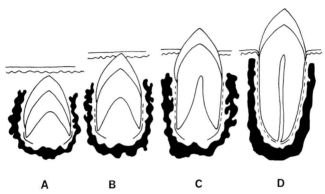

A   B   C   D

Fig. 76.—Four stages in the development and eruption of a tooth. During stages A, B, and C the tip of the lengthening root is maintained at the same distance from the lower border of the mandible. Alveolar bone develops around the erupting tooth. While the tooth erupts Hertwig's root sheath is pulled coronally together with the moving root. When the crown meets the opposing tooth the root begins to extend back into the jaw.

sheaths remain slightly separated in the region of the junction narrow dentine bridges connecting adjacent roots may be formed.

It will be recalled that when discussing the blood-supply to the tooth it was shown that vessels entering the dental papilla collect in groups whose number and disposition predict the location of the definitive roots. These groups of vessels lie in the bays in the developing root diaphragm, and the tissue tongues expand inwards between the vessels to unite in the less vascular centre of the crown base.

In single rooted teeth the procedure is precisely the same but no bays form in the free edge of the root diaphragm, probably due to the absence of developing lobes in the dental papilla. Furthermore, pulpo-periodontal canals are less common in the coronal half of these teeth.

Once the secondary apical foramina have been delineated in a multi-rooted tooth, a true Hertwig's sheath is present. This continues to grow in a vertical direction. The length of the root is a function of either the degree of intrinsic growth of Hertwig's sheath or of growth of the dental papilla and it is not yet conclusively established which tissue plays the dominant role.

As Hertwig's sheath grows vertically, it induces the differentiation of odontoblasts at the papilla surface. The odontoblasts produce the dentine of the root which lengthens in an apical direction.

After completing its organizing function, Hertwig's sheath fragments, remnants persisting in the adult periodontal ligament as the epithelial cell rests of Malassez. Various functions have been ascribed to these cell rests from time to time, though without any evidence. Histochemical studies reveal the continuing viability of these cells throughout life, albeit in a quiescent state so that the term 'rests' is a reflection of their metabolic state. The following suggestion is offered to explain the fragmentation of Hertwig's root sheath. It was noted that during the formation of the bud, cap, and bell stages of tooth development the free margin of the enamel organ (the cervical loop) grows around the expanding dental papilla. It has been demonstrated by serial radiographic examination that the tip of a growing root does not penetrate far into the basally adjacent alveolar bone until the tooth has erupted into the oral cavity and met its opponent (*Fig.* 76). Because the tip of the growing root is roughly stationary then so also is the tip of Hertwig's root sheath. In other words Hertwig's root sheath is not growing downwards into the jaw but the root dentine (and enamel) are moving away from it (*Fig.* 76A, B, C). As the cells of the root sheath proliferate in their continuing attempt to surround the dental papilla they may be pulled towards the oral cavity by the moving root. Because it is being pulled coronally by the lengthening root the proliferating root sheath is prevented from growing round the base of the papilla and sealing the apical foramen. The pull produces tension on the sheet of epithelial cells splitting it into a fenestrated pattern. This may explain why no degeneration of root-sheath cells is seen when it breaks up. When the erupting tooth has met its opponent the lengthening root can no longer slide past the root sheath which will now start to encircle the base of the papilla and complete the formation of the apical foramen of the tooth (*Fig.* 76D).

Although in Hertwig's sheath the cell layer nearest the papilla is directly continuous with the inner enamel epithelium over the crown, its cells do not pass through the same cycle of histodifferentiation, nor do they normally produce any enamel. The histochemical content of the two cell strata is different. Commonly, however, small enamel pearls are formed on the surface of roots, particularly at the bifurcation of roots. This shows, therefore, that some root-sheath cells are potentially capable of producing enamel. It is well known that coronal odontoblasts differentiate under the influence of the overlying inner enamel epithelium. There is no doubt that a similar inductive function is the prime role of Hertwig's sheath.

Unsuccessful attempts have been made to correlate the number and location of the roots with the position of the major cusps on the crown of the molariform tooth. In the late 18th century it was suggested that a relationship existed between the pattern of blood-vessels supplying the developing tooth and the presence of morphogenetic fields within it. More recently, these fields have been equated with cuspal areas, thought to be controlled by growth centres located within the pulp, under the influence of which specific parts of the crown pattern are generated. Direct evidence of these areas and centres is lacking, but it seems reasonable to expect that each should receive an adequate blood-supply via the roots. Hence the number and disposition of the roots would bear a relationship to the number and location of the cuspal areas and growth centres within the papilla, thereby establishing a link between the crown pattern and the root pattern.

REFERENCES

CARLSON, H. (1944), 'Studies in the Role and Amount of Eruption in Certain Human Teeth'. *Am. J. Orthod.*, **30**, 575.

GAUNT, W. A. (1960), 'The Vascular Supply in relation to the Formation of Roots on the Cheek Teeth of the Mouse', *Acta anat.*, **43**, 116.

KENNEY, E. B., and RAMFJORD, S. P. (1969), 'Cellular Dynamics in Root Formation of Teeth in Rhesus Monkeys', *J. dent Res.*, **48**, 114.

LESTER, K. S. (1969), 'The Incorporation of Epithelial Cells by Cementum', *J. ultrastruct. Res.*, **27**, 63.

NOBLE, H. W., CARMICHAEL, A. F., and RANKINE, D. M. (1962), 'Electronmicroscopy of Human Developing Dentine', *Archs oral Biol.*, **7**, 395.

ORBAN, E., and MUELLER, E. (1929), 'The Development of the Bifurcation of Multirooted Teeth', *J. Am. dent. Ass.*, **16**, 297.

SELVIG, K. A. (1963), 'Electronmicroscopy of Hertwig's Epithelial Sheath and of Dentine and Cementum Formation in the Mouse Incisor', *Acta odont. scand.*, **21**, 175.

CHAPTER XIX

THE PERIODONTAL LIGAMENT

THE periodontal ligament is a specialized connective tissue adapted to support the tooth in its bony socket and is derived from the dental follicle. Classically the 'dental follicle' is described as all the tissue between the forming alveolar bone and the forming tooth. However, if early stages of tooth development are examined it can be clearly seen that the ectomesenchyme of the dental papilla continues around the cervical loop of the enamel organ to form an investing layer around the developing tooth (*Fig.* 77). From this layer the cement forming cells are derived and it has been proposed that the term 'dental follicle' should be reserved for this investing layer rather than all the tissues between the tooth germ and the

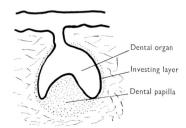

Fig. 77.—Diagram showing the continuity of the dental papilla with the investing layer around the dental organ.

surrounding bone. This contention is supported by evidence from culture studies. When tooth germs are permitted to survive in culture for thirty days, only a few scattered epithelial and ectomesenchymal cells remain. If these few cells are harvested and transferred to connective tissue of a host animal, they form a tooth germ surrounded by a dental follicle with, significantly, cement formation.

The main fibre groups of the functional periodontal ligament are adequately described in the literature and their anatomy is not considered here. Suprisingly little is known about the development of these main fibre groups. It has been suggested that the principal oblique fibres are orientated at the time of root development, an arrangement which is initially seen as an oblique orientation of fibroblasts synthesizing collagen which becomes alined along the same plane as the cells. However, this is by no means certain and it is also claimed that the development of oblique fibre groups does not occur until the tooth bears an axial load after eruption.

The configuration of the oblique fibres would suggest that they function as ties uniting the root to the alveolus and that under load these fibres transmit the force as tension to the alveolar bone. Indeed the oblique fibres are classically described as having a wavy configuration in the relaxed state but that they straighten out under load. However, there is now a great deal of evidence which shows that this concept is too simplified. For example, if the fibres of the periodontal ligament are cut on the mesial and distal aspects of the tooth, little increase in horizontal mobility occurs indicating that the fibres are not important in resisting horizontal force. Frequently, when dried skulls are examined, fenestrations in the labial wall of the alveolus not associated with pathological lesions are seen indicating that a complete bony alveolus is not necessary for tooth support. Under axial load it has been shown that the bony margins of the socket supporting the tooth dilate. If this axial load were converted to tension on the socket wall, as suggested by the orientation of the fibres, the reverse would be anticipated. This finding can be explained if a compressional system, as well as a tensional system, plays a significant part in tooth support. The ligament can be considered as a compressive hydraulic buffer consisting of a vascular component and a tissue fluid component. The suggestion is that, under axial compression, occlusion of the vascular elements occurs followed by the displacement of tissue fluid. However, it has been shown that the periodontal vessels of the monkey incisor unexpectedly failed to collapse when measured pressures were applied to the tooth and it has been suggested that the maintence of the patency of blood-vessels under pressure is a function of the oxytalan fibres found in the periodontal ligament. Oxytalan fibres are considered to be a variant of elastic tissue and have been shown to have a distribution within the periodontal ligament closely linked to blood-vessels. Thus they are found to run obliquely between vessels and cement, mainly perpendicular to the occlusal plane and at right angles to the direction of the collagen. The insertion of oxytalan fibres into cement implies an anchorage for the vessels which may permit them to accommodate distortion and compression strains.

The second component of this postulated hydraulic buffer mechanism, the tissue fluid, is considered to be more significant in terms of tooth support. As fluids are incompressible, the cells and extracellular fluid must be displaced if a tooth is pushed into its socket. Where the fluid is displaced is not known; it probably varies with the type of force. If the tooth is subjected to a horizontal force there is some degree of tilt and fluid can be displaced from a region of compression towards a region of tension. Under axial load the fluid can be displaced through the socket wall which is extensively perforated by foramina distributed mainly in the cervical and apical thirds. Also the outward displacement of the socket margin under axial compression suggests tissue fluid displacement towards the rim of the socket. In this case the collagen fibres act as ties preventing over dilatation of the socket.

A curious feature of the periodontal ligament is the persistence of the fragmented remnants of Hertwig's epithelial root sheath in the form of a network, the epithelial cell rests of Malassez. These persistent epithelial cells in the periodontal ligament serve no known function and indeed are not found in some species. In the rodent these cells are absent, the fragmented root-sheath cells being incorporated in the forming cement. In man the epithelial cell rests have been shown to be viable in the mature ligament and to have the histochemical and ultrastructural features of resting cells. It has been shown *in vitro* and *in vivo* that they retain their ability to divide and migrate under altered environmental conditions and form the epithelial lining of dental cysts.

Another controversial feature of the periodontal ligament is the existence of the so-called 'intermediate plexus'. The concept here is that in the middle region of the ligament the collagen of the principle fibre bundles is constantly being broken down and reformed to permit tooth movement in an occlusal direction. It has been argued that the histological demonstration of an intermediate plexus may be caused by the different planes occupied by the fibre bundles in longitudinal section of the tooth in situ. No intermediate plexus can be demonstrated in cross-sections through the ligament. However, although the bright field light microscopic appearance of an intermediate plexus may be artefactual, polarized light microscopy indicates that the collagen fibres in the central zone of the ligament are less mature. Also, in experimental avitaminosis C, which interferes with collagen production, the intermediate zone of the ligament shows the greatest degree of disruption which suggests that this is the most active site of collagen synthesis. Radiobiological studies have not helped as much as might have been anticipated. Studies, using radioactive proline, have not been able to demonstrate turnover in a clear cut intermediate zone. Instead a fairly even pattern of turnover occurs with the lowest activity towards the cement surface of the tooth.

The periodontal ligament, in addition to its main supportive role, has an important role as a sensory receptor. The ligament contains nerve-fibres running from the apical region towards the gingival margin which are joined by fibres entering the ligament laterally through the foramina of the socket wall. The latter divide into two, with one branch running apically and the other gingivally. The manner in which these nerve-fibres terminate is by no means certain. Small fibres are considered to terminate as fine arborizations and to be associated with pain. Larger fibres have been described as terminating as 'knob-like' endings, 'elongated' and 'spindle-like' endings, 'Meissner-corpuscle-like' endings, and 'irregular branched' endings. This variety of structural forms for nerve-endings in the ligament have been equated with the sensation of touch. They correspond in some degree to skin receptors. It has recently been suggested that these structural variations of the mechanoreceptors are not important but rather that their spatial arrangement within the ligament is the determining factor in their response characteristics. Overall they probably play a very important part in the control of mastication. Together with receptors in the muscles of mastication, the condyle, and the surface of the oral cavity they provide the 'input' to a centre in the cerebellum which reflexly controls the masticatory cycle. However, obviously the motor cortex has an over-riding control of this reflex centre. The blood-supply of the ligament is dealt with in Chapter VIII.

REFERENCES

ANDERSON, A. A. (1967), 'The Protein in Matrixes of the Teeth and Periodontium in Hamsters: A Tritiated Proline Study', *J. dent. Res.*, **46**, 67.

ANDERSON, D. J., HANNAM, A. G., and MATHEWS, B. (1970), 'Sensory Mechanisms in Mammalian Teeth and their Supporting Structures', *Physiol. Rev.*, **50**, 171.

BIRN, H. (1966), 'The Vascular Supply of the Periodontal Membrane', *J. periodont. Res.*, **1**, 51.

CARMICHAEL, G. C. (1968), 'Observations with the Light Microscope on the Distribution and Connexions of the Oxytalan Fibre of the Lower Jaw of the Mouse', *Archs oral Biol.*, **13**, 765.

CARNEIRO, J., and FAVA DE MORAES, F. (1965), 'Radioautographic Visualization of Collagen Metabolism in the Periodontal Tissues of the Mouse', *Ibid.*, **10**, 833.

ECCLES, J. D. (1964), 'The Development of the Periodontal Membrane in the Rat Incisor', *Ibid.*, **9**, 127.

GRUPE, jun., H. E., TEN CATE, A. R., and ZANDER, H. A. (1967), 'A Histochemical and Radiobiological Study of *in vitro* and *in vivo* Human Epithelial Cell Rest Proliferation', *Ibid.*, **12**, 1321.

HINDLE, M. O. (1967), 'The Intermediate Plexus of the Periodontal Membrane', in *Mechanisms of Tooth Support: A Symposium* (ed. ANDERSON, D. J., EASTOE, J. E., MELCHER, A. H., and PICTON, D. C. A.), p. 66. Bristol: Wright.

MAIN, J. H. P. (1966), 'Retention of Potential to Differentiate in Long Term Culture of Tooth Germs', *Science, N.Y.*, **152**, 778.

MUHLEMANN, H. R., and ZANDER, H. A. (1954), 'Tooth Mobility (III). The Mechanism of Tooth Mobility', *J. Periodont.*, **25**, 128.

PARFITT, G. J. (1967), 'The Physical Analysis of the Tooth Supporting Structures', in *Mechanisms of Tooth Support: A Symposium* (ed. ANDERSON, D. J., EASTOE, J. E., MELCHER, A. H., and PICTON, D. C. A.), p. 154. Bristol: Wright.

PICTON, D. C. A. (1965), 'On the Part Played by the Tooth Socket in Tooth Support', *Archs oral Biol.*, **10**, 945.

—— (1967), 'The Effect on Tooth Mobility of Trauma to the Mesial and Distal Regions of the Periodontal Membrane in Monkeys', *Helv. odont. Acta*, **11**, 105.

—— (1969), 'The Effect of External Forces on the Periodontium', in *The Biology of the Periodontium* (ed. MELCHER, A. H., and BOWEN, W. H.), pp. 363–421. New York: Academic.

TEN CATE, A. R. (1965), 'The Histochemical Demonstration of Specific Oxidative Enzymes and Glycogen in the Epithelial Cell Rests of Malassez', *Archs oral Biol.*, **10**, 207.

—— (1969), 'The Development of the Periodontium', in *The Biology of the Periodontium* (ed. MELCHER, A. H., and BOWEN, W. H.), pp. 53–90. New York: Academic.

ZWARYCH, P. D., and QUIGLEY, M. B. (1965), 'The Intermediate Plexus of the Periodontal Ligament: History and Further Observations', *J. dent. Res.*, **44**, 383.

CHAPTER XX

TOOTH ERUPTION

THE mechanism whereby a tooth moves through its surrounding tissues as it erupts is not yet fully understood. In consequence several theories of tooth eruption exist each involving the separate tissues of the dento-alveolar complex. During the past five years, however, there have been a number of studies which strongly implicate the periodontal ligament as providing the force for tooth eruption. Because some of these studies have provided negative results, in the sense that they have not directly shown involvement of the periodontal ligament but have eliminated other theories of tooth eruption, it is necessary to discuss these theories before finally discussing the role of the periodontal ligament in tooth eruption.

Root formation involves epithelial proliferation, dentine formation, and pulpal proliferation. Each of these, separately and together, has at one time or another been thought to provide the force for tooth eruption. Epithelial proliferation was thought to provide an axial force in the same manner as epithelial cells associated with growing hair. The continuation of tooth eruption after experimental removal of Hertwig's root sheath shows that epithelial proliferation cannot be considered as providing the force for tooth eruption. Furthermore, the fragmentation of the root sheath occurs relatively early in development of the tooth and epithelial proliferation could not, therefore, provide a sustained force of eruption. The formation of the root is linked with proliferation of the pulp cells and the growth of this tissue has been thought to provide a force sufficient to move the tooth. However, when democolcine is used to prolong the interphase stage of cell division, no effect on the eruption rate can be detected. Triethylene melamine destroys rapidly dividing cells. Its introduction into an experimental animal results in the complete loss of cellularity in the original proliferative area beneath the enamel organ and enclosed by Hertwig's root sheath. Such extreme cellular damage fails to halt tooth eruption, although the rate is slowed. Linked with root forma tion is the theory of pulpal constriction. This theory supposes that the progressive decrease in volume of the pulp cavity by continuous dentine formation results in the generation of a pulpal force through the apical foramen, akin to the thrust of a rocket. However, hypophysectomy, which results in increased dentine deposition and, therefore, increased constriction of the pulp, causes a slowing in the rate of tooth eruption.

When root formation is considered as a single entity, incorporating epithelial proliferation, dentine deposition, and pulpal proliferation, it is suggested that the increase in length of the forming root provides the eruptive force by the root pushing against a structure termed the 'cushion hammock ligament'. This structure was described as passing from one side of the socket, under the root apex, to the opposite wall of the socket and its function was thought to be to convert the downward force exerted by the growing root into a tensional component acting on the socket wall. It has now been clearly demonstrated that this structure is an artefact (*Fig.* 78) and is really a pulp delineating membrane with no connexion to the bone of the socket wall (*Fig.* 79). In addition, it has long been known that almost rootless teeth can erupt and that the length of the eruptive path of the human upper canine exceeds the length of the root. Significantly, in experiments, discussed in detail later, where the normal formation of the periodontal ligament is disrupted and tooth eruption halted, root growth continues with the result that the root buckles in the socket. This finding alone eliminates root growth as providing the force of tooth eruption.

Dentine   Cement

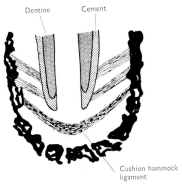
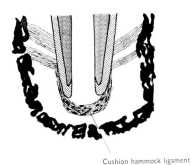

Cushion hammock ligament

Cushion hammock ligament

Fig. 78.—Diagram showing the location of the 'cushion hammock ligament'.

Fig. 79.—Diagram showing the correct interpretation of the so-called 'cushion hammock ligament'.

The vascular theory of tooth eruption suggests that the numerous blood-vessels in the apical follicular tissue maintain a relatively high extracellular fluid pressure in this confined area and that it is this pressure which provides the eruptive force. Experiments designed to increase and decrease the blood-flow are known to increase and decrease the rate of tooth eruption respectively. These experiments, however, only modify the rate of blood-flow and it does not follow that there will be a corresponding change in tissue fluid pressure. It is more likely that the changes in rate of eruption measured in these experiments are the result of changes in the metabolic activity of the periapical tissue.

A more critical experiment has recently been undertaken to determine whether or not capillary pressure, and therefore tissue fluid pressure, can be correlated with the rate of tooth eruption. Hypotensive drugs have been used to create a 20 per cent reduction in arteriolar pressure. Surprisingly, this degree of reduction in systolic blood-pressure is found to invoke an equivalent increase of pressure in the capillaries of the ear. The assumption is made that a similar increase in capillary pressure will be present in the periapical tissues. As there is no alteration in the eruption rate compared with that of the control animals, it is concluded that there is no basis for the vascular theory of tooth eruption. Finally, the eruptive force has been measured and has been shown to be of the order of 5 g., which is in excess of that which could be generated by tissue fluid pressure.

Bony remodelling of the jaws has also been linked with tooth eruption. It is suggested that the inherent growth pattern of the mandible or maxilla moves the teeth by selective deposition and resorption of bone in the immediate neighbourhood of the tooth. Elegant and careful studies with tetracyclines as bone markers disprove this theory. Tetracyclines become incorporated in newly formed bone and can be identified in sections due to their fluorescent properties. With the onset of tooth eruption there is bone resorption at the base of the socket. However, this is followed by deposition of bone on the socket floor and measurements have been made which show that the amount of bone deposited, plus the amount of root growth, together equals the distance the tooth moves. Although this finding would seem to implicate bone growth with tooth eruption, the initial resorption of bone as the tooth begins to move in an occlusal direction argues against bone providing any force. It is more likely that the later deposition of bone is an infilling after the tooth has moved.

Thus far all the studies which have been discussed show that the tissues of the forming root, the vascular elements, and bone are not capable of providing an eruptive force. The only remaining tissue which could provide an eruptive force is the follicular connective tissue and there is now positive evidence implicating this tissue in this role. Unlike previous theories of tooth eruption which involve the generation of a force to push the tooth from its socket, the tissues of the forming ligament are thought to pull the tooth into occlusion. Either the cells of the ligament or the extracellular collagen are thought to provide the force for tooth movement. In the forming ligament active collagen synthesis is taking place. It is assumed that as the fibroblasts secrete the tropocollagen macromolecules they are initially arranged in a random fashion in the extracellular compartment. These macromolecules now become ordered to form collagen (there is a decrease in entropy). There must exist a force along the axis of the orientating fibres which prevents the macromolecules from returning to their disordered state. A reasonable analogy here is a stretched elastic band. When stretched the molecules are in an orderly state (decreased entropy) and there is a contractile force as the molecules try and assume a more disordered state. Also, as the tropocollagen molecules aggregate to form collagen fibrils by the development of covalent cross-linkages, a contraction of about 10 per cent is thought to occur plus a further contraction due to dehydration. Thus, during collagen fibre formation a tensional force may develop, (1) due to decrease in entropy by electrostatic attraction of disordered tropocollagen molecules, (2) by linear polymerization producing a decrease in length of macromolecules, and (3) by shrinkage due to dehydration. The cells of the forming ligament may also provide a force akin to the contractile force which has been demonstrated in the healing wound. Although in this situation the cell has been directly implicated, rather than the collagen of the scar tissue, the manner in which the cell provides the force is not known.

At the present time experimental evidence implicates the collagen of the forming ligament rather than the cells. Chemical substances called 'lathyrogens' exert a specific effect by disturbing the formation of collagen; the formation of cross-linkages between the macromolecules of tropocollagen, and within the tropocollagen, is prevented. Administration of lathyrogen to experimental animals severely retards the eruption of teeth. When sections are prepared it is found that the architecture of the forming ligament is disrupted. Significantly, root formation is not affected and the growing root impinges on the floor of the socket with resorption of bone and buckling of the root. Also growth of Hertwig's root sheath is undisturbed and the predentine of the root, the pulpal tissue, and the vascular elements appear normal. Thus, the experimental prevention of normal collagen formation in the ligament prevents tooth eruption. It may be asked why it is that in this situation only the collagen of the forming ligament and not the collagen of the forming dentine of the root and alveolar bone is affected. It appears that there is a significant difference between soft tissue collagens and hard tissue collagens and that this difference lies in the nature of the cross-linkages. There is no direct experimental evidence which might implicate the cells of the ligament at this time. However, no matter whether the force of eruption is a property of forming collagen or of the cells of the ligament, there can be no doubt that the forming ligament is responsible for the force of tooth eruption. A very elegant experiment unequivocally shows this to be so. If the continuously erupting rodent incisor is transected and an artificial barrier placed between the two components, the following results. The distal portion of the tooth continues to erupt and is eventually exfoliated. This portion of the tooth cannot have moved due to forces generated by root growth, blood-pressure, or apical bone growth as these factors have been eliminated. Only the periodontal ligament remains. The proximal portion of the tooth continues to grow and because the artificial barrier prevents tooth movement, the apical tissues extend backwards within the bone of the jaw. This one experiment clearly points to the tissues of the periodontal ligament providing the force for tooth eruption.

It must be noted that the above theory depends almost entirely on evidence obtained from the continuously erupting rodent incisor. However, it seems reasonable to assume that a similar mechanism is involved in the eruption of human teeth.

REFERENCES

BERKOVITZ, B. K. B., and THOMAS, N. R. (1969), 'Unimpeded Eruption in the Root-resected Lower Incisor of the Rat with a Preliminary Note on Root Transection', *Archs. oral Biol.*, **14**, 771.

JENKINS, G. N. (1966), *The Physiology of the Mouth*, 3rd. ed. Oxford: Blackwell Scientific.

MAIN, J. H. P. (1965), 'A Histological Survey of the Hammock Ligament', *Archs oral Biol.*, **10**, 343.

— — and ADAMS, D. (1966), 'Experiments on the Rat Incisor into the Cellular Proliferation and Blood-Pressure Theories of Tooth Eruption', *Ibid.*, **11**, 163.

NESS, A. R. (1964), in *Advances in Oral Biology* (ed. STAPLE, P. H.), vol. 1, 33–70. New York: Academic.

TEN CATE, A. R. (1969), 'The Mechanism of Tooth Eruption', in *The Biology of the Periodontium* (ed. MELCHER, A. H., and BOWEN, W. H.), pp. 91–103. New York: Academic.

CHAPTER XXI

THE DENTO-EPITHELIAL JUNCTION

THE attachment of the gingiva to the tooth is a natural weak point in the integument of the mouth and is the site of onset of many periodontal lesions. Because of this the dento-epithelial junction has been the subject of intensive investigation during the past few years and our understanding of this area has much improved. To understand the histology of this attachment apparatus, and to discuss the problems associated with it, it is best to begin with an account of its development. Briefly stated, as the

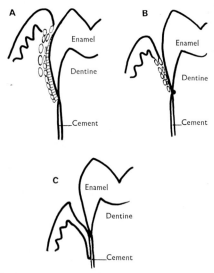

Fig. 80.—Diagram showing the change in the attachment with age. A, As the tooth erupts the attachment consists of dental and oral epithelium. B, Attachment at the cement-enamel junction C, Attachment on the cement surface.

tooth erupts the reduced enamel epithelium covering the occlusal surface fuses with the oral epithelium. With continued eruption cells from this combined source, now termed the 'epithelial cuff', migrate apically over the reduced enamel epithelium covering the sides of the crown and, for a time, these combined epithelial layers constitute the epithelial attachment. With further eruption of the tooth the enamel epithelium component is lost and the epithelial attachment then consists only of cells derived from the cuff, and extends as far as the cement-enamel junction. In time the attachment gradually migrates onto the cement covering the root. It is evident, therefore, that the nature of the attachment not only varies as the tooth erupts into the oral cavity but also with age (*Fig.* 80).

Before describing the epithelial attachment of the gingiva to the tooth in detail it is helpful to consider the way epithelial cells are joined to each other and also the way in which an epithelium is attached to its supporting connective tissue. The manner in which epithelial cells join each other is by means of the desmosome. This structure consists of components contributed by the two cells in contact with each other (*Fig.* 81). As the cell membrane approaches the region of contact its two layers, as seen with the electron microscope, thicken considerably. The cytoplasm on the inner

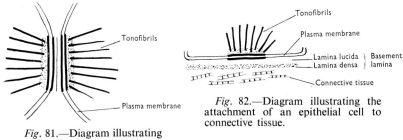

Fig. 81.—Diagram illustrating the desmosome.

Fig. 82.—Diagram illustrating the attachment of an epithelial cell to connective tissue.

aspect of this thickened part of the plasma membrane is more electron dense and numerous tonofilaments radiate from this electron-dense cytoplasm. This structural arrangement is repeated in the adjacent cell and, in the narrow gap between the two cells, a fine electron dense line can be distinguished (Chapter II).

Where an epithelial cell is in contact with connective tissue the electron microscope shows that the epithelial cell has hemi-desmosomes (*Fig.* 82) which represent half a desmosome. In addition two further layers are seen: a lamina lucida and a lamina densa together termed the 'basement lamina'.

At the time the attachment consists of reduced enamel epithelium and the migratory epithelium from the cuff, there is no argument that a true attachment exists. The reduced enamel epithelium consists of two cell layers. An inner layer consisting of reduced non-formative ameloblasts and an outer layer of polygonal cells probably derived from the stratum intermedium of the dental organ. The reduced ameloblasts are attached to the enamel surface by means of hemi-desmosomes and basement lamina in the same way that epithelial cells elsewhere are attached to their supporting connective tissue. The reduced ameloblasts are joined to the cells of the outer layer by means of desmosomal attachments. In turn the epithelial cells migrating apically over the reduced enamel epithelium have been shown to develop desmosomal attachments with the outer layer cells of the reduced enamel epithelium (*Fig.* 83).

At the time the last edition of this book was being prepared there were conflicting opinions concerning the precise nature of the epithelial attachment when the enamel epithelial component is lost. The nature of this attachment has now been elucidated with the aid of the electron microscope. The epithelial cells adjacent to the enamel surface possess hemi-desmosomes and are in contact with a basement lamina just as at any other epithelial connective tissue junction. In addition, a cuticular layer is interposed between the basement lamina and the tooth surface which is thought to represent accumulated basement lamina material (*Fig.* 83). The epithelial nature of this attachment can be amply demonstrated by removing the attached gingiva and thoroughly curetting the epithelium from the tooth surface. Within two months a new attachment forms featuring hemi-desmosomes and a basement lamina. When the epithelial attachment occurs on the cement surface instead of the enamel, the attachment is still seen morphologically as consisting of hemi-desmosomes and a basement lamina.

Although the nature of the epithelial attachment is now understood, there are still some intriguing problems associated with the attachment

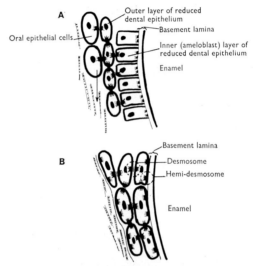

Fig. 83.—Diagram illustrating the differing nature of the epithelial attachment. A, With the reduced dental epithelium. B, Without reduced dental epithelium.

apparatus which require discussion, especially with respect to the provision of an adequate seal between the external environment and the underlying connective tissue.

If we again consider the situation just before the tooth breaks through the oral epithelium it is apparent that there is a removal of connective tissue over and surrounding the crown of the tooth. Electron microscopic studies of physiological connective tissue resorption in this region have shown that, until the tooth breaks through the oral epidermis, this connective tissue breakdown involves fibrocytes and macrophages. As soon as the tooth breaks through the oral epithelium, a classic inflammatory response occurs within the connective tissue, evidenced by the accumulation of polymorphonuclear cells. This inflammatory response at this time in tooth eruption has also been demonstrated in gnotobiotic (germ-free) animals. The occurrence of an inflammatory lesion at this time implies the failure of the developing attachment to provide an adequate barrier to the oral environment. Significantly it has been shown that with continued tooth eruption and further development of the epithelial attachment, repair takes place simultaneously with breakdown in the connective tissue supporting the developing attachment.

There are many reports in the literature of an interdependence between connective tissue and its overlying epithelium and that one feature of epithelium associated with disturbed connective tissue is the presence of large intercellular spaces between the epithelial cells. These spaces provide a potential pathway for antigens through the epithelial cells which, in turn, could lead to the persistence of a localized inflammatory area beneath the epithelium of the attachment. Indeed, this inflammatory focus is regarded as a normal feature of this area by many investigators. Whether material is capable of passing inwards through the epithelium of the attachment apparatus is still not settled. Certainly material can pass outwards. A simple experiment demonstrates this. If the gingival sulcus in an experimental animal is sealed with an acetate film, and the sulcus examined histologically some days later, it is found to be filled with cellular detritus derived from the viable attachment and with a fluid exudate. Evidence is now accumulating which suggests that material can also pass inwards. In the fully erupted tooth it has been shown that carbon particles penetrate through the crevicular epithelium covering inflamed tissue. Tritiated thymidine has also been shown to penetrate crevicular epithelium of the fully developed attachment. Significantly when tritiated thymidine is dripped over the cusp of a monkey tooth whose cusp had just broken through the oral mucosa, labelling is found in the connective tissue cells supporting the developing attachment, indicating the ability of small molecules to penetrate the forming attachment at the time of tooth eruption. Thus there is the strong possibility that the attachment is not an impenetrable barrier and therefore the initiation of periodontal disease may occur at the time the tooth breaks through the oral epithelium.

REFERENCES

ENGLER, W. O., RAMJFORD, S. P., and HINIKER, J. J. (1965), 'Development of Epithelial Attachment and Gingival Sulcus in Rhesus Monkeys', *J. Periodont.*, **36**, 44.

LISTGARTEN, M. A. (1967a), 'Electron Microscopic Study of the Gingivo-dental Junction of Man', *Am. J. Anat.*, **119**, 147.

— — (1967b), 'Phase Contrast and Electron Microscopic Study of the Junction between Reduced Enamel Epithelium and Enamel in Unerupted Human Teeth', *Archs oral Biol.*, **11**, 999.

— — (1968), 'Electron Microscopic Features of the Newly Formed Epithelial Attachment after Gingival Surgery. A Preliminary Report', *J. periodont. Res.*, **2**, 46.

— — (1970), 'Changing Concepts about the Dento-epithelial Junction', *J. Can. dent. Ass.*, **36**, 70.

STALLARD, R. E., DIAB, M. A., and ZANDER, H. A. (1965), 'The Attaching Substance between Enamel and Epithelium. A Product of the Epithelial Cells', *J. Periodont.*, **36**, 130.

TEN CATE, A. R. (1971), 'Physiological Resorption of Connective Tissue associated with Tooth Eruption and Electron Microscopic Study', *J. periodont. Res.*, in the press.

Chapter XXII

THE FINAL INVESTMENTS
OF THE CROWN OF THE TOOTH

As sometimes happens electron microscopy not only reveals hitherto unobserved structures but also results in interpretations of structures that are quite different from those made by light microscopy. The prism sheaths in enamel were one example of this and the cuticles of the tooth are another. It is convenient to start with the interpretations of the light microscopists.

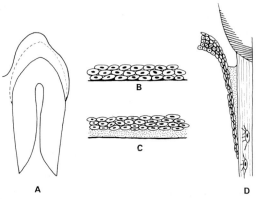

Fig. 84.—When a recently erupted tooth is dissolved in acid a membrane floats from the surface of the dissolved enamel (Nasmyth's membrane, A). This consists of the reduced enamel epithelium and possibly a thin inner structureless layer, the primary enamel cuticle (B). Sometimes a much thicker structureless layer, with different staining properties, intervenes between the two layers (secondary enamel cuticle, stippled in C), although the primary cuticle indicated in this diagram is usually not seen. A secondary enamel cuticle (stippled in D) may also separate the cement from the epithelial attachment.

In the last century the two-layered appearance of a membrane which covers newly erupted teeth was described (*Fig.* 84A, B). The outer layer of this membrane is cellular and probably consists entirely of the remnants of the enamel organ which covered the fully developed enamel. For obvious reasons this cellular layer is called the 'reduced enamel epithelium'. The inner layer, about whose presence there has been disagreement, is about 1μ thick, is not always seen, and has a structureless refractile appearance. It is called the 'primary enamel cuticle' and is perhaps the partially mineralized or unmineralized last formed product of the ameloblasts.

Occasionally, beneath the reduced enamel epithelium, there is present a considerably thicker structureless layer (about 4μ thick) which stains in a characteristically different way from the somewhat refractile primary enamel cuticle (*Fig.* 84C). This is called the 'secondary enamel cuticle' and has been considered to be secreted by the reduced enamel epithelium rather than by the ameloblasts *per se*. A similar cuticle can often be seen between the cement and the epithelial attachment (*Fig.* 84D). This has been considered to be secreted by the cells of the epithelial attachment when they have grown on to the surface of the cement. The primary enamel cuticle of the crown, and the secondary enamel cuticle of both crown and root region have been considered to be of importance in cementing epithelium to the tooth surface.

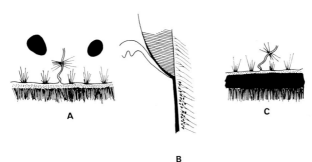

Fig. 85.—A primary enamel cuticle may exist only over the cervical enamel. It appears to be continuous with, and similar in structure to, the cement (B). Enamel crystallites are separated from the reduced enamel epithelium by a basement membrane (stippled in A) and 'joined' to it by hemi-desmosomes. Where a primary enamel cuticle is present a basement membrane also separates it from the reduced enamel epithelium (C).

The primary enamel cuticle has recently been studied by electron microscopy. The most surprising aspect of this work was the finding that, apart from in the region adjacent to the cervical enamel (*Fig.* 85B, C), the light microscopist's primary enamel cuticle was not present. Instead, a basement membrane about $\frac{1}{10}μ$ thick (and therefore beyond the resolution of the light microscope) separated the surface enamel crystallites from the cells of the reduced enamel epithelium (*Fig.* 85A). It was therefore suggested that the primary enamel cuticle of the light microscopists is an artefact produced by light being in some way interfered with by the inner cytoplasm or cell membranes of the reduced enamel epithelium. However, it must be remembered that many light microscopists had already considered that the primary enamel cuticle was not always present. It may be that, because in electron microscope studies relatively few specimens are investigated as compared with the numbers investigated in light microscope studies, material containing a primary enamel cuticle has not yet been studied by electron microscopists.

The cells of the reduced enamel epithelium are joined to the basement membrane by a desmosome-like structure. Because the desmosomal elements are confined to one cell (instead of the usual two adjacent cells) the structure is referred to as a hemi-desmosome (*Fig. 85A, C*). In passing, it is worth noting that the elements of the basement membrane in this situation must be entirely derived from cells of ectodermal origin (*compare* Chapter II).

In a similar study of the root surface a secondary cuticle, equivalent to that of the light microscopists, was observed. It has not yet been observed by electron microscopists on the crown of the tooth. Nevertheless, the light microscopists finding that a secondary cuticle may exist on the crown of a tooth was not disputed. At present the light microscopists have suggested two possible origins for the secondary enamel cuticle. First, it may be a physiological product of the adjacent epithelial layers and be

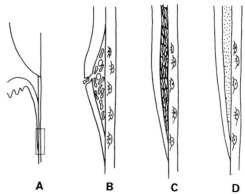

Fig 86.—Possible mode of formation of the secondary enamel cuticle in the root region of a tooth. Boxed region in A is shown in B, C, and D.

concerned with cementing the epithelium to the tooth surface. Second, it may have a pathological origin (*Fig. 86*). Blood-cells from small haemorrhages in the tooth follicle or periodontal ligament may leak through the epithelial layers lifting either the reduced enamel epithelium or the epithelial attachment away from the surface of the tooth (*Fig. 86B*). The blood-cells autolyse and iron becomes reabsorbed back through the epithelial layers (*Fig. 86C*). The larger molecular weight proteins break down but are not reabsorbed and remain, what is in effect, outside the body (outside the epithelia). Here they condense together becoming the secondary enamel cuticle (*Fig. 86D*). Particularly convincing has been the demonstration that a layer of red blood-cells squashed on to a wax surface can produce *in vitro* a structure which resembles in all ways a secondary enamel cuticle.

Other integuments found on the surfaces of teeth are food debris, dental plaque which consists of a soft mass of bacteria, and cellular debris which accumulates rapidly in the absence of oral hygiene, and finally calcified deposits on the tooth surface (calculus).

These integuments do not really concern us here. They are, however, of great importance in the onset both of carious lesion and of periodontal disease.

REFERENCES

DAWES, C., JENKINS, G. N., and TONGE, C. H. (1963), 'The Nomenclature of the Integuments of the Enamel Surface of Teeth', *Br. dent. J.*, **115**, 65.

HODSON, J. J. (1966a), 'The Distribution, Structure, Origin and Nature of the Dental Cuticle of Gottlieb, Part I and Part II', *J. Am. Soc. Periodont.*, **5**, 237, 295.

— — (1966b), 'Electron Microscopic Study of the Gingivo-dental Junction of Man', *Am. J. Anat.*, **119**, 147.

LISTGARTEN, M. A. (1966), 'Phase-contrast and Electron Microscopic Study of the Junction between Reduced Enamel Epithelium and Enamel in Unerupted Human Teeth', *Archs oral Biol.*, **11**, 999.

CHAPTER XXIII

AGE CHANGES IN THE DENTAL TISSUES

IN animal wildlife teeth are such important structures that the loss of the dentition marks the end of an animal's life-span. Although this is not true of modern man the teeth exhibit senescent phenomena which are important. Perhaps the most important age changes are the wear of enamel (because it cannot be replaced) and the apical retreat of the epithelial attachment (which must eventually lead to the loss of the tooth).

Enamel is a relatively inert tissue because it has no cellular component. However, certain age changes take place in response to attrition and to physico-chemical changes in structure.

The most conspicuous age change associated with enamel is its loss due to wear. This loss is extremely variable depending on the diet of the individual, the nature of the occlusion, and the composition of the enamel. Attrition of the occlusal surfaces of teeth is obvious. Attrition also occurs at the contact points between teeth due to the differential movements of adjacent teeth during mastication, and the extent of this wear can be considerable. It has been estimated that by the age of 40 as much as 1 cm. can be lost from the overall circumferential length of the arch in the average complete dentition.

The use of dyes and radioactive isotopes has shown conclusively that enamel is slightly permeable, and that this permeability decreases with age. It seems that ions are exchanged between the surface enamel and saliva. It is well known that fluorine is most beneficial if the ion is incorporated within the enamel during its development, or absorbed onto its surface immediately after its appearance in the oral cavity. The reduction of the incidence of caries in young individuals exposed to fluoride can be explained by the higher permeability of younger enamel to ions. There is little evidence for any change in the organic content of the enamel with age and this is not surprising in view of the nature of this non-vital tissue. Thus, it can be stated that the changes that are brought about in enamel with increasing age are those of a physico-chemical nature, and result from the interaction between the oral environment and the enamel surface.

Age changes in the dentine are more marked because, unlike enamel, this tissue is vital. The formation of dentine continues throughout life but at a diminishing rate, so that the volume of the pulp chamber progressively diminishes. Recent studies have shown a marked difference in the composition of the matrix of the rapidly formed primary dentine compared with the slowly formed physiological (or regular) secondary dentine. In addition to the deposition of this secondary dentine, dentine is also deposited in response to advancing attrition and dental disease. In response to these stimuli pathological (or irregular) secondary dentine, in which a reduced number of tubules pursue a haphazard course, is deposited. Physiological secondary dentine would appear to be a natural consequence of ageing unrelated to injury of the tooth.

Another age change in dentine, not necessarily related to the pathology of the tooth, is the formation of translucent or sclerotic dentine. Here the tubules of the dentine are progressively occluded, by deposition within their lumens of mineral salts, so that the now mineralized tubules have the same refractive index as inter-tubular dentine. It is thought that the tubules become filled with peri-tubular dentine. Although translucent dentine can develop anywhere in the dentine, it is consistently found in the root region after middle age. Teeth containing translucent dentine appear to be more brittle than other teeth making them more liable to fracture during extraction.

Dead tracts are also found in dentine. Here the odontoblast process degenerates leaving an empty tubule. Such tubules are, however, sealed off at their pulpal end by the deposition of pathological (irregular) secondary dentine. When viewed in transmitted light dead tracts appear more opaque than normal dentine due to the presence of air in the empty tubules. Although translucent dentine and dead tracts frequently form in response to attrition or dental disease, there is ample evidence that both changes can be independent of peripheral injuries, and they must consequently be regarded as progressive age changes within dentine.

Cement is deposited intermittently throughout life around the roots of teeth and there is a loose correlation between the thickness of cement and age. This relationship is a linear one, but the thickness of cement is too readily influenced by the functional stresses applied to the tooth and by periodontal disease, to provide a wholly reliable indication of dental age.

With the initial completion of the apex of the root the dental pulp can be considered to have attained maturity. The pulp has been shown to be similar in composition, organization, and histochemical reactivity to other connective tissues, and it bears the same relationship to dentine as bone-marrow to mineralized bone. Functionally, pulp and dentine should be regarded as the two parts of one tissue and in consequence some of the age changes of dentine are also age changes of the pulp.

The young pulp contains many fibroblasts, young collagen fibres, and relatively few mature collagen fibres, all disposed in a fluid ground substance. With advancing age, mature collagen fibres increase in number, cellular elements decrease, and the ground substance becomes less aqueous. These changes may be the result of a diminishing blood-supply to the pulp consequent upon vascular strangulation by narrowing of the apical canal and upon progressive arteriosclerosis. It is also claimed that the nerve-supply to the pulp diminishes with increasing age.

Radiographs often reveal the presence of mineralized nodules within the pulp cavity of the tooth. Under the light microscope these 'pulp stones' can have one of two appearances. Either the irregularly mineralized nodules may contain a few randomly arranged tubules or they may have the appearance of a relatively acellular bone. The first type is called a true pulp stone (because it contains 'dentinal tubules'), the second a false pulp stone. With the progressive deposition of dentine on the walls of the pulp cavity these stones may finally become embedded on the encroaching pulpal surface of the dentine. Another variety of ectopic mineralization is referred to as 'diffuse calcification of the pulp'. In this case irregular strands (rather than discrete nodules) of poorly mineralized tissue are found distributed throughout the pulp. The origin of pulp stones is unknown. Perhaps following a minute pulpal haemorrhage, extravasated blood-cells form a focus for the development of fibrous tissue which subsequently becomes mineralized. Layers of mineralized tissue are now deposited around this focus to form the discrete mineralized nodule. But this cannot explain the presence of 'dentinal tubules' in a pulp stone. It will be recalled that odontoblasts are only differentiated under the influence of the internal enamel epithelium or Hertwig's root sheath and neither of these is present in the pulp. Diffuse calcification of the pulp is probably produced in response to the decreased vascularity of an ageing pulp but the mechanism by which it is produced is not known.

The periodontal ligament forms the attachment between tooth and bone and the life span of the tooth depends upon its integrity. Little is known of the quantitative and qualitative changes occurring with age within the ligament itself except that it may become narrower with age; far more attention has been paid to the apical downgrowth of the epithelial attachment with age. Two opinions have been expressed in attempts to explain the cause of the retreat of the attachment. Some consider it is a direct response to inflammatory change in the periodontal ligament, and it is true that in sections of this region some evidence of inflammatory cell infiltration can always be found. An alternative interpretation is that the retreat of the attachment is a physiological process termed 'passive eruption'. In other animals, where gingival disease is not as widespread as in man, slow gingival recession proceeds as an apparently normal age change and this fact has been used as an argument against the belief that inflammatory change is the causative factor.

Whatever the reason for the retreat of the attachment, it will be appreciated that it must be preceded by the removal of the adjacent gingival fibres of the periodontal ligament and be followed by resorption of the bony alveolar crests. Finally, even if it is accepted that regression is related to age, this does not necessarily mean that this is a physiological ageing process. Taking all the evidence into account, it is most likely that it is the environment of the attachment which results in its downward retreat with age.

Clinical observations give the impression that the oral mucosa in the aged is thinner, dryer, and more fragile. However, little work has been done on this problem; such work is urgently required because of its clinical significance. What evidence there is suggests that there is diminution in keratinization with age, but this has been obtained from studies involving cytological smears which at best are capricious.

Studies of teeth have proved exceptionally useful in determining the age of mutilated or otherwise unrecognizable bodies. It is obvious that up to the age of twenty the developing and erupting teeth provide an accurate estimate of an individual's age. However, even beyond this time teeth frequently provide very good estimates of age. Longitudinal ground sections of a single tooth or several teeth are prepared. The following five features are studied: attrition, secondary dentine, translucent dentine, the position of the epithelial attachment, and the thickness of the cement. Each of these features is given a score from 0 to 3. Zero represents the condition expected in a perfect young tooth whereas 3 represents an extremely advanced stage of, for instance, spread of translucent dentine, attrition, or cement thickness. The five scores are added together to give a final figure. Thus a single tooth may score attrition 2, secondary dentine 1, translucent dentine 3, epithelial attachment 1, cement 2. The total is 9. By referring to published tables a good estimate of the age of a person having teeth with a score of 9 can be obtained.

REFERENCES

BERNICK, S. (1967), 'Age Changes in the Blood Supply to Human Teeth', *J. dent Res.*, **46**, 544.

BLACK, G. V. (1924), in *Operative Dentistry*, 6th ed. vol. 1, p. 223. London: Kimpton.

GUSTAFSON, G. (1950), 'Age Determinations of Teeth', *J. Am. dent. Ass.*, **41**, 45.

JENKINS, G. N. (1966), *The Physiology of the Mouth*, 3rd ed., pp. 157, 241. Oxford: Blackwell.

MILES, A. E. W. (1961), 'Ageing in Teeth and Oral Tissues', in *Structural Aspects of Ageing* (ed. BOURNE, G. H.). London: Pitman.

— — (1963), 'The Dentition in the Assessment of Individual Age in Skeletal Material', in *Dental Anthropology* (ed. BROTHWELL, D. R.). Oxford: Pergamon.

PHILLIPAS, G. G., and APPLEBAUM, E. (1966), 'Age Factor in Secondary Dentine Formation', *J. dent. Res.*, **45**, 778.

ZANDER, H. A., and HÜRZELEGER, B. (1958), 'Continuous Cementum Apposition', *Ibid.*, **37**, 1035.

130

INDEX